50

MISCONCEPTIONS OF

SEX

A MODERN
TANTRIC PRACTICE

Alexa Vartman

50 Misconceptions of Sex
A Modern Tantric Practice
First Edition. V.1

Copyright © 2020 by Alexa Vartman.
Book and cover design: Matías Baldanza.

Printed in the United States of America

First Printing, 2020

ISBN # (Ebook): 978-1-8380056-2-7
ISBN # (Paperback): 978-1-8380056-0-3
ISBN # (Hardcover): 978-1-8380056-1-0

TNT Education
71-75 Shelton Street, Covent Garden
London WC2H 9JQ, ENGLAND

This book uses British conventions for spelling and grammar, including the usage of single quotation marks.

*In dedication to my teachers and mentors,
without whom this book would not exist.*

DISCLAIMER

This book details the author's personal experiences with and opinions about tantra and sexuality. The author and publisher are providing this book and its contents on an *'as is'* basis and make no representations or warranties of any kind with respect to this book or its contents. The author and publisher disclaim all such representations and warranties. In addition, the author and publisher do not represent or warrant that the information accessible via this book is accurate, complete or current.

The information provided in this book is designed to provide helpful information on the subjects discussed. This book provides content related to tantra and sexuality. As such, use of this book implies your acceptance of this disclaimer.

You understand that this book is not intended as a substitute for consultation with a licensed healthcare practitioner, such as your physician. This book is not meant to be used, nor should it be used, to diagnose or treat any medical condition, sexual issue, trauma or mental health issue. For diagnosis or treatment of any medical problem, sexual issue, trauma or mental health issue, consult your own physician or another licensed healthcare practitioner.

Before you begin any new practice, or change your lifestyle in any way, you should consult your physician or another licensed healthcare practitioner to ensure that you are in good health and that the examples contained in this book will not harm you.

The publisher and author are not responsible for any specific needs that may require medical supervision and are not liable for any damages or negative consequences from any treatment, action, application or preparation, to any person reading or following the information in this book. References are provided for informational purposes only and do not constitute endorsement of any websites or other sources. Readers should be aware that the websites listed in this book may change.

THANK YOU

Gabriela Maya Mesquita, for the cover photo make-up and for guiding me so eloquently in my female exploration and growth.

Marieke Drost, for tirelessly checking all the references.

Ladybug, for the great creative writing.

Sandi Smith, for all the proofreading.

Apollo, for the very valuable guidance and scientific/philosophical commentary and always keeping my feet on the ground.

And most of all to Paris Cecilia Jayer, for keeping me going with this project in difficult times. What would I do without you?

Cover photo credit: Jan Dahlqvist, Asfalt Communication AB.
Best photographer eva!

Please excuse my average writing skills. I was only ever a C+ English student at school, but I know these teachings have the power to change people's lives for the better. So bear with me as I struggle to try and keep your attention and hopefully give you a modern and practical guide to modern Western tantric practices and enough footnotes and scientific references for credibility.

P.S. I don't recommend reading this book if you don't have a sense of humour.

CONTENTS

CONTENTS

FOREWORD

My wish list of people that I would love to write this foreword:

Ru Paul
Lana Wachowski
Elizabeth Gilbert
Caitlyn Jenner
Stephen Fry
Angelina Jolie
Esther Perel

1

YOU DON'T NEED A BOOK TO LEARN SEX

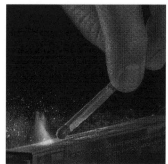

Advanced Sex 101

'Draw!' —she yells through her freshly applied lip gloss, as both men fumble to undo their trousers.

'Ready your weapons' —she says with a naughty smirk, while she skilfully inserts her black nails into her G-string and slides it down to just above her knees… I can see she is enjoying this, already.

I look on nervously, as I let out a barely audible laugh and my easily amused mind starts entertaining a silly thought: *'This brings a whole new meaning to the phrase cockfighting!'*

Allow me to start a few fires inside the fragile sexual egos of men, and introduce this book with a good old-fashioned poke in the eye with a blunt stick!

Tantric Yore

In the olden days of years gone by, there were mythical tantra practitioners who claimed they could do wonderful and mysterious things that regular men could not. Things like giving a woman a full body orgasm from 20 feet away, a womb orgasm that lasted for 20 minutes at a time, a cervix orgasm, and also satisfy a fair maiden for an entire weekend.

Their techniques were shrouded in mystery to protect the flailing members of mere mortal men who lived shackled by instant gratification.

While many of these so-called experts claimed to be skilled tantric practitioners to allure fresh interns, the truth was that *most* of them were inept in their art; they were simply not up to the task. As a consequence, the board of the Tantric Monks devised a devious plan.

To sort out the men from the charlatans, they inaugurated an annual Tantric Monks and Harlots Showdown. Instead of *'Pistols at dawn'*, they had *'Dicks at dusk'*. Instead of duellists shooting each other to draw blood from a newly drilled orifice, they selected a few trusted women (with naturally occurring and much more willing orifices) for the participants to unleash their tantric carnal prowess on. At the end of the showdown, the female jury would determine, without a doubt, which tantric master was the real deal and which had put themselves into the now embarrassing position of self-proclaimed (and now, obviously deluded) tantra teacher.

Just to keep the stakes high (and to add insult to injury), the winner would take all the loser's students (and thus, their source of livelihood) and disappear into the forest with a new entourage of freshly invigorated fair maidens, not unlike the fabled pied-piper.

Or something like that...

Now I know most people think a master lover is someone who *'copulates like a porn star on amphetamines with a rather oversized member,'* but that's not entirely true, old boy! In fact, it's not even close. The problem is that we simply don't have credible knowledge about expert lovers in our society. Let me try and explain... hopefully, without getting a hatchet thrown at my head.

Most men operate on about 5 to 10% of their full sexual energy (and potential) because, instead of building up their most valuable, creative, life energy and use it as a gift to their lover or to fuel their creative projects, they waste it by clenching their lower body to extract the instant-gratification thrill of a 5-second spasm orgasm, collapse into a heap, and finally wonder why their partner just got less attractive. Pizza anyone?

There's a whole new world of sex out there. A world that operates with different laws of (sexual) physics that was hidden for ages in tantric monasteries. A world that now is beginning to reveal itself to the modern man. This world is full of unknown phenomena such as many different kinds of tantric orgasms, methods that allow the penis and vagina to feel each other without needing friction, that sex *can be* pleasurable for hours without losing energy (or interest), and that women can have pain-free orgasmic births, to name just a few.

Luckily, none of the secrets revealed in this book is beyond the reach of the average Joe or even takes years to master. So, men; here is my invitation to you. Follow the simple instructions in this book, and you'll be well on your way to becoming one of the rare and few men that women chase. Not because you have a fat wallet, or because you look like George Clooney or have Brad Pitt's irresistible smile. I'm talking about becoming a *master lover*. The master lover is a scarce breed who lives in a world where the tables have been turned. How many average-looking men do you know that get paid by women to have sex with them? It's a great job if you can get it!

So, by all means, apply these techniques to become a better person and gift your sexuality to the world. My hope is that you don't make the mistake of misusing these techniques as *'party tricks'* to inflate your sexual ego. Instead, I hope you use your newly acquired swag to make this world a little better. From my perspective, it could use some sprucing up.

However, before we get into the nuts-and-bolts, I must come clean. I have a hidden agenda for writing this book. I don't have a tantrically skilled boyfriend. It gets kinda weird with men that have been to one of my workshops as they automatically see me as the alpha, and I'm doing my darnedest to be the passive beta. So, here I am, joining the global feminine cry from every pram-filled café around the globe: *'Where are all the good men?'*

In this book are the sexual teachings from one of the longest-running, biggest, most notorious, scariest, wildest, craziest and certainly most controversial tantra organisations in the world, without having to take your clothes off and attend one of their highly-confrontational workshops. (Or, God forbid, have to meet face-to-face with their weirdo founding father? Umm. Mother? Err. Whatever I am)[1]

---

1. Reading this first chapter, you might get an idea of why I got the name *'provocateur'*. It goes both ways, you know... you poke, you get poked back. If you're the kind of person with an annual subscription to *People Magazine* and love gossip, drama and good old-fashioned name-calling, then checkout my *'colourful'* reputation. The executive summary is that I've been called many charming names from *'psycho cult leader'*, *'sexual predator'* to an *'energy sucking lizard alien'* and *'perverted weirdo'* (this one, I don't contest though) by my critics... who mainly consist of envious disgruntled ex-employees (and now business competitors) who all seem to have one trait in common: they previously revered/idolised me waaaay too much! Witnessing how accusations without evidence can be used to justify hateful judgement of those peculiar to the herd, gives me first

So, to conclude my little pre-ramble...

In honour of the tantric showdown, I publicly challenge all other tantra schools in the world to a tantric shindig against the top tantric gigolos of The New Tantra (TNT). Duh, da duh! Just to sort *'those who can'*, from *'those who think they can'*. And I'll be watching... with my skirt hitched high. While I have never heard any reports from the roaming workshop junkies of a stronger form of tantra practitioners out there, if there is one I want to be one of the first to know it, so I can learn it and copy it, like so many have done to us. At least in Europe, the majority of new tantra schools appearing over the last 10 years have been past students of TNT. As they say, *'emulation is the greatest compliment'*.

Photo credit: *Yann Segalen, https://commons.wikimedia.org/wiki/File:Friction_d%27une_allumette.jpg UNDER [CC BY-SA 4.0 (https://creativecommons.org/licenses/by-sa/4.0/)]*

---

hand experience of Rene Girard Mimetic Theory of Scapegoating. Ah, the joys being even a tiny bit famous in these days of social media and dealing with a controversial topic like sex! Otherwise, if you feel that indulging in the *'he-says-she-says'* is beneath your level of dignity, or if you don't really care because you have next to no chance of hanging with me in person, then let's get to the good stuff that might actually change your life for the better. For more information about Mimetic Theory, you can refer to https://woodybelangia.com/what-is-mimetic-theory/

2

THE CLITORIS IS THE WOMAN'S BEST FRIEND

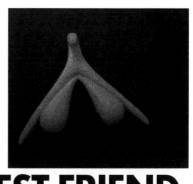

The Pudendal Nerve Caution

Men got a bit of a bashing in the last chapter, so now it's the turn for women to receive a little ruffling of their feathers (and in the interest of self-preservation, I will tread far more cautiously).

The old song proclaiming *'diamonds are a girl's best friend'* may be highly contested on a lonely, cold and dark night. For the less financially inclined women, clitoral orgasms might be the best 5 to 10 seconds of the day. And why not? It is relatively easy to achieve, can be an effective sleeping aid and stress reliever, plus it feels damn good... (Or so I'm told. I didn't get one of those with the dress.)

Women have rightfully fought long and hard at educating men about the exact location of their little love button and the proper stimulation techniques, so I think I'd better be careful about saying anything even appearing to be negative about the clit or I might get a slap in the face with a wet vibrator. If you're interested in the female genital anatomy, please check these footnotes.[1,2]

Over the years, I've met thousands of women in my workshops with similar stories of sexual shame. Often their conservative upbringing suppressed their sexual needs, but then one glorious day, they discovered their clitoris. Some, with a pillow squeezed between the legs, or the

---

1. https://www.teenvogue.com/story/vagina-anatomy-diagrams
2. https://www.academia.edu/22796305/Anatomy_of_the_Clitoris

shower-head in the bath. Others perhaps a little finger wiggle while they fantasised about naughty things.

I'm all for women having as many orgasms as they desire. However, in a tantric sense, there are more intense and longer-lasting orgasms than the clitoral orgasm.[3] When a woman orgasms in this way, it can be similar to the male ejaculation orgasm. A relatively brief and intense orgasm, but in the female's case, can be linked together in a chain of orgasms. For most sexually active women, clitoral orgasm is part of the regular sex diet. But what if there were better options?

Here's a testimonial from a female TNT workshop participant:

During my twenties and even in my thirties, I had a sort of a sexual heyday. On any given Friday or Saturday night, you would find me either picking up some beautiful person at the club or on a date with my current sweetheart. I didn't worry about the sexual abilities of the person I was with, I just picked them based on how sweet they were or how good-looking. Their sexual skill didn't matter so much because I knew how to make myself cum. Everything seemed fine, but I did have a nagging feeling that there had to be some-thing better.

I stumbled onto tantra at a time when I didn't think I really needed it and wasn't even expecting to learn anything transformational. I was resistant to the teachings of avoiding cumming with my clit because that was an easy way to get off and the only way that had consistently delivered the most intense results for me.

I completed the 21-day challenge[4] (of not orgasming with the clitoris) as an experiment, and what I found was that once my pussy was de-armoured (in the TNT level 2 workshop), I could enjoy more intense sex and orgasms in different ways. Now I can experience longer, more intense orgasms when my pussy is relaxed and not tense from frequent orgasms on my clit. The orgasms that I have been routinely having from deep penetration with a toy or a cock have been worth the annoyance of giving up my daily clitoral orgasm regime.

The Pudendal Nerve

Many female tantric practitioners have expanded their repertoire of orgas-mic possibilities and generally agree that there are longer-lasting, deeper

---

3. https://medicalxpress.com/news/2009-09-vaginal-orgasm.html
4. www.21daychallenge.com

and more satisfying orgasms than the clitoral orgasm that operates through the pudendal nerve.

Unfortunately, like so many things in life that are worth doing, there is a learning curve and a price to be paid. The price is that to have the deeper tantric orgasms, most women need to discipline themselves to give up the clitoral orgasm, either temporarily or permanently.

To understand why it's often necessary to trade one for the others requires some insight into the inner workings of the woman's body, so let's start at the top (so to speak). The brain is connected to the clitoris via the pudendal nerve. This is the same nerve that connects a man's brain to his penis. (Yes, there actually *is* a brain-to-penis connection, thank you ladies!) This nerve provides a pathway that can trigger a *'peak'* orgasm. Interestingly enough, *'Pudendal'* is Latin for *'to be ashamed of'*. Great! So, does this mean we've been orgasming on the shame nerve?

Pudendal nerve orgasms are similar in both men and women, and there is a reason for this. In the embryonic stage, the clitoris and the penis are anatomically the same, so they share the same neural pathways. In fact, when people describe their experience of orgasming on the pudendal nerve without reference to genitals, their descriptions are indistinguishable.

- They both can relieve stress.
- They usually last for about 5-10 seconds.
- They are accompanied by a pumping sensation/spasms/contractions in the genitals.
- After one or more of these orgasms, the level of horniness generally diminishes.

Because of the build-up and crescendo effect of the regular orgasm, the rhythmic contractions and brief nature associated with the pudendal nerve, in 2011 I devised the term *spasm orgasm* to be used interchangeably with *peak orgasm* to differentiate the regular pudendal nerve orgasm from tantric orgasms that do not have these qualities.

Most of us are familiar (in one way or another) with male ejaculation followed by losing arousal/energy/interest and finally falling asleep after climax. The recovery time to become ready for sex again is called the *sexual refractory period* and is typically more pronounced with men. The refractory period varies significantly among women. While some women describe their own post-orgasmic period in a similar way to men, others do not. Women can be interested in orgasming a few times before they stop, but eventually *'La petite mort'* (the little death) will rain on the sexual parade. If this weren't the case, our teenage urges would probably have kept us thrashing around down there until our hands were worn to a nub! Whilst men in particular may be familiar with the sexual hand-brake after orgasm, the science to explain exactly what happens after orgasm is still not completely clear.

The refractory period (MRP) continues to be a topic of discussion and debate within the field of sexual medicine.[5]

One plausible theory seems to be that ejaculation creates a pressure loss in the seminal ducts, and this triggers a signal that temporarily halts sexual appetite, but this is obviously only relevant to men. Another theory that encompasses both genders is that progesterone spikes after climax and triggers a loss of sexual appetite.[6]

Clitoral Hiatus

Back to that *price* I mentioned earlier. I'm not trying to railroad you down the path of better sex and a healthier, more sustainable sex life :) Everyone is free to do with their bodies what they want; but if you choose to learn the other tantric orgasms (which we will cover later in this book), it will be necessary to put clitoris stimulation on a temporary pause.

According to my scientist friends (in the unfortunate position of having to explain brain physiology to me in layman's terms), the clitoris *screams* a loud signal to the brain. This signal overrides other neural pathways that could produce other orgasms if they weren't overwhelmed by that noisy little pudendal nerve. I guess this is like trying to hum a song when another tune is playing loudly in the background. Indulging regularly in this type of orgasm makes the brain highly attuned (and even addicted) to that signal.

Conditioning of response exclusively to clitoral stimulation interferes with the development of vaginal feeling. —Arnold Kegel in *'The Journal of the American Medical Association'* (1953).

Luckily, a period of clitoral abstinence allows the brain to re-map it's *listening* abilities and tune into other nerves that can orgasm more deeply, thanks to a process called *neuroplasticity*.[7] The price of admission into the

---

5. https://onlinelibrary.wiley.com/doi/full/10.1111/bju.12011

6. https://www.medicalnewstoday.com/articles/324887.php

7. https://en.wikipedia.org/wiki/Neuroplasticity

world of deeper tantric orgasms is to give neuroplasticity time to do its thing. And, yes, in practice this means giving up direct clitoral stimulation for an extended period of time — for example, one year. (Don't hate me, ladies. I'm just the messenger!) This will give the brain time to re-map itself to be able to orgasm on other nerves like the hypogastric, pelvic and vagus nerve.

Edging

Does that mean one should never, ever touch the clitoris again? No, not necessarily. There are more advanced techniques that can be learnt *after* mastering other tantric orgasms. The addiction to clenching and squeezing the bodily base can be transcended through the practice of *'edging'*.[8] Edging (or *OMing*)[9] is a bodily awareness/discipline technique that consists of stimulating the pudendal nerve but refraining from orgasm. One simply trains oneself to notice the habit of clenching to squeeze stimulation into a crescendo, and do the exact opposite—relax, breath regularly, keep your legs open and don't give in to the urge of grabbing the low-hanging fruit. Wait for 30 seconds, rinse and repeat. More on this later.

Photo credit:
Thelma Amaro Vidales (https://www.shutterstock.com/g/Thelma+Amaro+Vidales), https://www.shutterstock.com/image-photo/photo-close-pink-clitoris-plastic-clays-1399703735

8. https://www.sexcoaching.com/sexual-pleasure/edging-for-women/
9. https://www.healthline.com/health/orgasmic-meditation-101

3
EJACULATION IS DESIRABLE

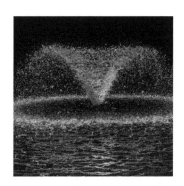

But is it Beneficial?

We probably all have a friend or relative with an annoying dog that loves to hump people's legs, right? Have you stopped to consider how often the dog ejaculates on its victim's pants? Sorry for graphic image, but the answer is virtually *never*. The really interesting question though is: *'why not?'* The same question applies to when a dog licks its genitals. Why doesn't it continue until climax like humans do, if it's so natural?

If, by *'natural'* we mean *'in alignment with other species unmodified by human behaviour,'* it seems that masturbation until ejaculation is *not* as natural as we commonly assume. Mankind is pretty much unique in the animal kingdom when it comes to routinely *'rubbing one out'* to the point of orgasm.

If I were to ask you which animal masturbates the most in the animal kingdom, you might get the unwanted flashback of a moment in the zoo, trying to look the other way when a monkey starts pleasuring itself in front of embarrassed parents — rapidly whisking their children off to a more suitable attraction. The other reasons that we often associate masturbating animals with primates is they are one of the few animals classified as *continuous breeders* — animals whose fertility is not limited to one or two seasons per year. Primates also masturbate in a way that reminds us of our own *'going it solo'* habits. But unlike humans, they rarely masturbate to climax.

A recent article in Scientific American described a 1983 study of wild grey-cheeked mangabeys in the Kibale Forest of Western Uganda. Scientists kept track of the sexual behaviour of several groups of primates over the course of 22 months. The mangabeys had plenty of sex and many of the males masturbated (especially when the females were at their most fertile), but the scientists only witnessed two occurrences of a male mangabey masturbating to the point of ejaculation in that entire time. (And I thought I had a strange job!) Both incidents happened when females were nearby and engaging in loud sex with other males.[1]

Other primate studies reported similar findings. In 2004, male red colobus monkeys were observed for a period of five and a half years, totalling 9,500 hours of observation, but only five incidents of masturbation to the point of ejaculation were recorded.[2]

It would seem that humans are rather unique in the animal kingdom in our masturbation ejaculation habits. Certainly, we ejaculate more frequently than what might be considered *natural* compared to non-human primates and the rest of the animal kingdom.[3]

Let's look more closely at humans. According to sexologist and zoologist Alfred Kinsey, in his landmark 1950 book *Sexual Behaviour in the Human Male*,[4] 92% of American males admitted to regularly masturbating to the point of orgasm. We assume that if a man masturbates, he is probably going to 'finish' unless he is interrupted or has some kind of medical problem that prevents him from ejaculating. It's so ingrained in our culture that anything less can be seen as abnormal, as described by the word 'anorgasmia'.

So, despite non-human primates having the capacity to masturbate to ejaculation, for some reason they don't. This begs the question: 'Why not, when doing so feels so good?' Perhaps the goal of sex is naturally different than hyper-orgasming humans assume?

The Goal?

Recent research carried out by the brilliant (and brave) sexual psychophysiologist Dr. Nicole Prause[5] shows that the biggest reason for having sex is of course pleasure, but new technology in measuring brain

---

1. https://link.springer.com/article/10.1007%2FBF02743755
2. https://www.ncbi.nlm.nih.gov/pmc/articles/PMC3810986/
3. https://blogs.scientificamerican.com/bering-in-mind/
   one-reason-why-humans-are-special-and-unique-we-masturbate-a-lot/
4. https://en.wikipedia.org/wiki/Kinsey_Reports
5. https://www.liberoscenter.com

stimulation using electroencephalography EEG[6] shows that the greatest reward (and associated motivating factor) for sex is actually the *high arousal state* during the act and *not* the 8-12 rhythmic contractions of the regular spasm orgasm. This has been found to be evident in both men and women.

Her research seems to support the tantric experience that the regular orgasm is really not as important as is commonly assumed for the overall joy of sex, especially if the arousal state is expanded, deepened and prolonged. It would be very interesting to have her conduct research on our tantric practitioners.

For a short summary of her work I highly recommend her insightful YouTube clip.[7]

Photo credit: *Rudy and Peter Skitterians* (https://pixabay.com/users/skitterphoto-324082/), https://pixabay.com/photos/fountain-splash-water-drop-scatter-2498605/

---

6. https://journals.plos.org/plosone/article?id=10.1371/journal.pone.0165646
7. https://www.youtube.com/watch?v=aK-zBBSqFV4

4

IT'S DANGEROUS NOT TO EJACULATE

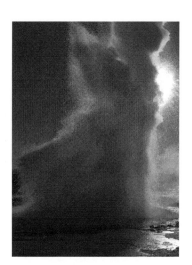

Sure About That?

Knowing most animals do not ejaculate nearly as often as humans do, the notion that not ejaculating is dangerous might not be as solid as it seems. An interesting observation in cross-species studies is that only people and dogs get *'naturally occurring'* prostate cancer in significant numbers.[1] In other words, prostate cancer is not observed at a rate even close to humans in most other animal species. The reason for this is unclear.

It seems most people (or, at least, most of the ones which I come in contact with) are familiar with a comprehensive study done in 2016 by Harvard Medical School on 32,000 men over the course of 18 years, which reported a 20% reduction in prostate cancer for men that ejaculated more than 20 times a month, compared to those who did so only four to seven times a month.[2] It would, therefore, appear that men should *'beat the meat'* to achieve better sexual health and that the whole tantric *not-ejaculating-thing* is dead in the water. Well, not so fast...

As I am not a scientist or a doctor, I will quote directly from the highly respected medical website WebMD's opinion about this study:

While research is promising, there's still a lot scientists need to learn.

---

1. http://www.animalresearch.info/en/medical-advances/diseases-research/prostate-cancer/

2. https://www.webmd.com/prostate-cancer/ejaculation-prostate-cancer-risk#1

Some things to consider:

- There's no proof that ejaculating more actually causes lower chances of prostate cancer. For now, doctors just know they're connected. It may be that men who do it more tend to have other healthy habits that are lowering their odds.
- Ejaculation doesn't seem to protect against the most deadly or advanced types of prostate cancer. Experts don't know why.
- Scientists don't know if ejaculation during sex vs masturbation has the same benefits. [...]
- Not all studies have found a benefit. The 2016 study got attention because of its size (almost 32,000 men) and length (18 years). But some smaller studies have not shown the same good results. A few even found that some men, specifically younger men, who masturbated more, had slightly higher chances of prostate cancer.

Although there are certain well-documented risk factors, according to the American Cancer Society: science and the medical profession still don't know *'exactly what causes prostate cancer'*.[3] In fact, even though prostate cancer is the second most common cancer in American men, with 1 in 9 men being diagnosed with prostate cancer, we know less about what causes it than we do about most other types of cancer in humans.[4, 5]

From the list above, I think the third bullet point is very interesting. Since the study did *not* include sex without ejaculation, one possible explanation is that sexual *pleasure in itself* (rather than ejaculation) causes a lower risk of prostate cancer.

Interestingly, there does not seem to be any scientific studies that provide any evidence that sexual abstinence is dangerous for the prostate. Anorgasmic males and virgin males who have never orgasmed do not report higher rates of prostate cancer.

My Personal Prostate Health

Some people assume that those who abstain from sex may be at risk of prostate cancer, but there is no evidence to support such a claim.

---

3. https://www.cancer.org/cancer/prostate-cancer/causes-risks-prevention/what-causes.html
4. https://www.cancer.org/cancer/prostate-cancer/about/key-statistics.html
5. http://www.irishhealth.com/askdoc.html?q=6873&qasect=11

Nevertheless, the study encouraged me to pay closer attention to the health of my prostate. I have been a tantric practitioner since 2000, and I want to be as sure as I can that I'm not endangering my own health and other men's health by recommending the practice of non-ejaculation.

Although there is no perfect test to detect prostate cancer, the best we have right now is the Prostate-Specific Antigen test or PSA.[6] I took the PSA test a few days ago, it came back at a nice low level. Better safe than sorry.

More Specific Studies, Please

What would really be helpful is a clinical study done on healthy, vital men who choose to never ejaculate but still masturbate and stay *sexually active*. I have never heard of such a study. Perhaps because there are not many tantric sexually active men who choose not to ejaculate to act as a control group. In the 2016 study, so few men ejaculated less than 3 times a month that the researchers had to disregard this data sample because it was too small. This might warrant further studies that *include* tantric men that rarely ejaculate but have the ability to circulate energy. It could be that the ability to circulate sexual energy as described in this book may be an important variable in this mystery.

Test It for Yourself

In this book, I'll show you how to try these things for yourself, and in a fairly short time, you might experience quite drastic changes in your physical abilities. You can try these techniques out as an experiment, and see if these practices work for you. I also recommend getting your PSA test done (regardless of your age), so you can have a baseline indicator of your current prostate health and verify if these tantric practices have any impact on it. Prevention is always preferable to cure.

Photo credit: *Hans Braxmeier* (https://pixabay.com/users/hans-2/), https://pixabay.com/photos/geyser-water-fountain-explosion-3242008/

---

6. https://www.cancer.gov/types/prostate/psa-fact-sheet

5

ORGASMS ARE ALL GOOD

Brain Chemistry and Mood

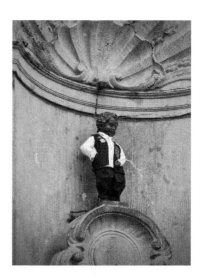

In general, life is better when you have a good sexual relationship. You'll get no argument from me about that. Research shows that sex is also good for the body, heart and brain.[1] However, it seems that not all orgasms have the same after-effects.

Believe me, I would love to preach the popular belief that the more orgasms of any sort, the merrier, but if you learn how to have more tantric orgasms you might notice that in contrast to the short, intense spasm orgasms, tantric orgasms leave very tangible long-term benefits. Please excuse this chapter if it gets a little geeky.

Post-Sex Blues?

While it doesn't seem to be a universal truth, many people notice a subtle delayed melancholic feeling after having a regular orgasm, either right away, or in the following days.

In 2009, Dr Richard A. Friedman, MD, writing for the health section of *The New York Times*, observed patients experiencing postcoital depression [PCD].[2] Dr Friedman noted that he found many online forums with people

1. https://health.clevelandclinic.org/why-sex-is-good-for-your-health-especially-your-heart/
2. https://www.nytimes.com/2009/01/20/health/views/20mind.html

discussing post-sex sadness. Even now, ten years later, a quick Google search shows that sadness after sex is not at all uncommon. In fact, in a study published in the *Journal of Sex & Marital Therapy* in 2018, of the 1,208 men surveyed, 41% of them admitted that they had experienced *'inexplicable feelings of tearfulness, sadness or irritability following otherwise satisfactory consensual sexual activity.'*[3] A similar study of women published in 2015 showed a similar statistic — 46% of the 230 women surveyed reported that they had experienced PCD. Researchers from the Queensland Institute of Technology have theorised that hormonal shifts occuring after orgasm could be to blame and that these serve evolutionary functions.[4] More on that in a minute.

In other words, some people (but certainly not all) report feeling sad and crabby over varying periods of time after pudendal nerve orgasms. On occasion, this can happen right after the orgasm, but also in post-orgasm days, making it more difficult to notice cause and effect. Once again, more research is required to connect these outcomes, but in the meantime, if you are interested in learning more about this, you have all the equipment to be able to test it for yourself. (That is, if you can discipline yourself enough to abstain for a while.) One female TNT workshop participant conducted such an experiment by herself in December 2019 and wrote a report on it:

I've been practicing tantric sex since 2012 which means I have purposefully stopped having clitoral orgasms for about 8 years at the point that I write this report. These days I only have a clitoral orgasm by accident a few times a year. I love my tantric practice and can't imagine ever going back to "regular" sex.

However, a few months ago, before the Christmas holidays of 2019, I wanted to do an experiment. It's been so long since I experienced any sort of "orgasm hangover" feeling or grumpiness after having clitoral orgasms, so I wondered how it would feel if I gave myself a few on purpose. That night I ended up giving myself 7 clitoral orgasms in a row and 2 more the next day.

Conclusion of this experiment:

1. *Wow, I can't believe people think this orgasm is so great. It feels only localized in one spot and every orgasm gets less and less intense after*

---

3. https://www.tandfonline.com/doi/abs/10.1080/0092623X.2018.1488326

4. https://www.dailymercury.com.au/news/
    why-almost-half-women-feel-sad-after-sex/2798936/

the last one. My tantric orgasms are much longer and pleasurable and I feel them deeper in my body. For the last few clitoral orgasms I had to rub intensely and contract my body so I could have the little explosion of pleasure. I almost broke out into a sweat! Not worth it, in my opinion.

2. *The next couple of days I felt like my head was coated in a thick cloud of grogginess. Almost as if my forehead was contracted into a hard ball. I felt so grumpy, antisocial and tearful for no reason. I didn't do any of the activities I had planned that day. My room mates said I was extremely hard to reach, as if I was "lost inwards", inside of my own head, instead of being engaged and present with the world outside of me.*

My take-aways from this experiment:

- *I'm certainly not going back to orgasming regularly on my clit. I feel so much better when I don't and my tantric practice is way more satisfying.*

- *If women give themselves clitoral orgasm every week, how can they know how it feels to not have these negative post-orgasmic feelings? I can't even imagine how it must feel for men. From observing my male lovers in the past, I feel like ejaculation has an even a stronger effect on them than the clitoral orgasm has on women.*

Rats!

According to scientists, rats are useful in human research because of the close correlation to lower-brain functions like sex (thanks!), as well as the ease of isolation of single variables. From research in rats by T. H. Krüger, the feel-good neurotransmitter *dopamine* drops below normal levels in both male and female rats after orgasm, and prolactin also appears to diminish sexual arousal after orgasm.[5] The findings from this study showed that when male rats have an infinite supply of female rats to copulate with (ie *hump till ya drop*), they became bored with the females for several days. In their study, it took up to 15 days for them to recover their sexual appetite.[6] I guess that females just don't look so appealing after you ejaculate so many times. At least for rats.[7]

A research from 2014 does seem to have shown that ejaculation, even

5. https://www.ncbi.nlm.nih.gov/pubmed/15889301

6. Phillips-Farfan and Fernandez-Guasti, 2009 https://www.ncbi.nlm.nih.gov/pmc/articles/PMC3319191/

7. https://www.reuniting.info/science/sex_in_the_brain

twice a week, shrinks the dopamine-producing neurons in the ventral tegmental area (a midbrain structure that is rich in dopamine neurons, part of the mesolimbic dopamine pathway and an important part of the "reward system."), which reduces a male's response to the pleasure of morphine.[8] This also happens with repeated heroin use in both rats and humans.

Although there is a lack of scientific evidence about post-orgasmic dopamine levels in humans (as few volunteers have come forth to have holes drilled their head), the prolactin spike is well-studied in cases of decreased sexual appetite in humans.[9] After ejaculation (and to varying degrees in females after regular spasm orgasms), the body produces serotonin, which in turn stimulates prolactin. In layman's terms, a spike of prolactin puts out the sexual fire.[10] Prolactin secretion seems to occur when men experience rhythmic contractions while ejaculating, even in *dry-orgasms*. This matches our experience that the contractions are the relevant factor in question and *not* the actual seminal fluid. This means that the lack of involuntary spasms allows sex to continue to be appealing despite seminal oozing (pre-come).

Due to the lack of data on this topic, this is also an area of sexology that would benefit further research.

Testosterone Influences Us All

If you've ever watched boxing movies or documentaries, you might be familiar with the scene where the coach warns the athlete not to have sex before the big game. From experience, they noticed that athletes will have less energy and be a little more lethargic after sex. While this seems to make some sense, why do some athletes and their coaches believe in the benefits of abstaining for a week before an athletic event? To answer this question, we must understand a little more about testosterone. The Journal of Zhejiang University has documented the strong testosterone spike that occurs after 7 days of abstinence following an ejaculation orgasm.[11] Another study by the Department of Life Science, Hangzhou, found evidence that testosterone levels increase by nearly 150%, after

---

8. https://www.ncbi.nlm.nih.gov/pubmed/24966382#
9. https://www.ncbi.nlm.nih.gov/pubmed/14656205
10. https://www.ncbi.nlm.nih.gov/pubmed/12697037
11. https://rd.springer.com/article/10.1631/jzus.2003.0236

abstaining for 7 days.[12] Testosterone has a strong impact on mood and sex drive on males, but it seems to affect both sexes.[13]

Since low testosterone is a common cause of depression in men,[14] it seems reasonable to try and observe how our habitual behaviours may be impacting our testosterone levels. Although ejaculation does not have an *immediate* impact on testosterone levels, the receptors that help the body utilise free testosterone — called *'androgen receptors'*, may be damaged by frequent overuse. A 2007 study on rats found that frequent orgasms lowered androgen receptors in their brains.[15] We are not rats, but we do have androgen receptors, and just like in rats, these receptors help our bodies use testosterone. This may explain correlated findings in humans.

There is a simple test to get your testosterone levels checked. Testosterone cream can give an ageing man his mojo back in a few days and make a big difference in mood, but only if his levels are low (less than 300 nanograms per decilitre). This might explain why ejaculation may have a greater negative long-term effect as mood depressor in ageing men, who already have lower testosterone levels. When we are young, we seem to be able to ejaculate and recover quite quickly. For most men, the refractory period increases with age.

Estrogen Isn't Only for the Ladies

A study by the Department of Pharmacobiology, CINVESTAV, México City, showed that frequent ejaculation increases estrogen receptors.[16] Estrogen receptors allow the body to utilise estrogen. So for men, excess estrogen in your body may increase the likelihood of developing those sexy man boobs, a round feminine belly, becoming more lethargic and reducing muscle mass![17] So, although sexual arousal and pleasure are positive things, over-indulging in the normal spasm orgasm may have side-effects that we

---

12. https://www.ncbi.nlm.nih.gov/pubmed/12659241

13. http://www.bumc.bu.edu/sexualmedicine/publications/
    testosterone-insufficiency-in-women-fact-or-fiction/

14. https://www.webmd.com/depression/news/20040203/
    low-testosterone-cause-depression

15. https://www.researchgate.net/publication/6536830_Relationship_between_Sexual_
    Satiety_and_Brain_Androgen_Receptors

16. https://www.ncbi.nlm.nih.gov/pubmed/17239879

17. https://www.healthline.com/health/masturbation-and-testosterone#research

didn't count on.

But, don't despair! Tantric orgasms through other nerves: hypogastric, pelvic and the vagus nerve don't cause these adverse effects. As such these tantric orgasms are considered *healthy* orgasms.

A Post-Orgasm Example

Different people notice different patterns after spasm orgasms. Here is the general pattern I've observed, although results vary quite considerably depending on many other factors. Most people won't notice trends unless they keep a mood journal to track cause and effect so I highly recommend doing so to be able to see how the regular orgasm may be affecting you:

- Immediately after ejaculation, I usually lose most of the previous horniness and interest in sex and may become more lethargic or sleepy. Physically, there may be a pleasant relaxation in the body, but sometimes there is also a subtle dull pain in the perineum.
- Over the next 3 days, there is little noticeable change. The physical refractory period can be quite short, and the potential to become interested in sex is still there.
- Between day 4 and 6, I notice a loss of sexual appetite and a some-what nasty, irritable grumpy mood can sometimes develop, making me have a generally shorter *'fuse'* toward my partner. This effect is not very noticeable if this was the first ejaculation in a long time, but negative effects seem to accumulate when several ejaculations have occurred in a short period of time. If it was the first ejaculation in many months, the effects could be barely noticeable, but multiple ejaculations can create a very noticeable *'orgasm hangover'*. (This is an easy experiment to try for yourself!)
- On day 7, the well-documented testosterone spike hits, as evidenced by the return of the *'early morning glory'*.
- Mood and overall energy levels improve progressively from day 10 to about 2 weeks after the orgasm. After that, there are no noticeable improvements in mood, subtle, relaxed horniness and energy. In general, I develop a subtle sense of well-being, greater patience and emotional resilience (especially in my relation to a sexual partner).

Try it out for yourself, but be aware that the more variation in your lifestyle during your *'sexperiment'*, the more difficult it will be to isolate one variable.

Check Out 21daychallenge.com

The New Tantra created a free website you can use to support your little experiment.[18] See if you can make it to 21 consecutive days without a pudendal nerve orgasm (both for men and women). However, you are welcome to stay sexually active with either intercourse or masturbation. In fact, it's better if you do so. Roughly 85% of people report that they don't go back to old habits once they see the benefits of this most basic tantric practice.

There is even some scientific suggestion that the production and usage of sperm consumes far more biological resources than has been previously assumed, and may account for the shorter lifespan of males compared to females. That's been found to be true for worms at least.[19]

Love Skills?

Regardless of whether you notice a change in mood and energy, one thing is pretty certain to happen: You will undoubtedly become more sexually sensitive, and this usually equates to being a better lover. You will be able to rely less on high-speed friction to feel sensations and will develop a greater ability to slow down and have a wider range of speeds, so you won't just have the one setting of *'the Energizer Bunny with a jackhammer'*. The ability to slow down becomes much more important for both men and women when they don't want to go careering over the *'point of no return'*.

However, the biggest impact on male sex prowess is that the spasm reflex to contract the bodily base (for the brief 5-second thrill) will be annoyingly close for about 10 days after ejaculating. For me, that meant that I could not follow the woman into her horniest tantric orgasms without losing control. She had to learn to restrain herself and not surrender completely... perhaps not the best scenario for aspiring tantric practitioners.

It would seem that improving your *'under the sheets stock price'* has a price: A little good, old-fashioned abstinence, sacrifice and self-discipline.

---

18. www.21daychallenge.com and sign up for free coaching on tantric sex.

19. The simple act of making sperm substantially shortens a male worm's life span, a researcher has discovered in results that overturn accepted biological dogma about the relative cheapness of a male's ejaculation compared with the preciousness of a female's egg. The scientist studying simple but revealing worms called *'nematodes'* found that males live much shorter lives than their mates, and he has traced that discrepancy to sperm production. —*The New York Times*, December 3, 1992

ORGASMS ARE ALL GOOD

Tantra uses the lure of sex to motivate practitioners to do intense renunciation and bodily meditation practices.

Photo credit: *Ji-Sun Yoo* (https://pixabay.com/users/ssalae-369698/), https://pixabay.com/photos/brussels-europe-belgium-1017986/

6

NO EJACULATION = BLUE BALLS

Bollocks!

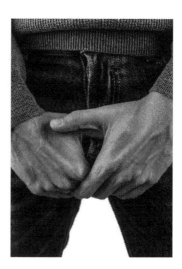

'Blue balls' is the common expression for the mild pain in the testes that appears after a few days of not ejaculating, or after sexual arousal without release. When first practising non-ejaculation tantra, many men *do* experience the *'jewels in the velvet vise'* somewhere around day 10 after their last ejaculation. The good news is that I've never heard of it continuing indefinitely.[1]

There is a medical name for it; it's called *epididymal hypertension*. The pain is caused by blood vessels expanding as they re-acclimatise to your pre-pubescent, pre-ejaculation days. Probably, ever since the first time you learned to orgasm, all your horny episodes sent blood rushing to your genitals, which was then followed by a rapid outflow of blood after ejaculation. The result of this is that your body is trained to expect only short-term arousal and release. It takes a week or two for the body to get back to how it was before you joined the frequent ejaculation program with *'Madam Palmer and the 5 sisters'*. (Masturbation that is gents.)

The other technical name for blue balls is also not so sexy, *Vasocongestion*. Think of it as a kind of traffic jam in your nuts, in which instead of cars trapped on a motorway, you have a higher genital blood pressure than you are used to. Some men even report a little blood in the semen the first

---

1. Please drop me a line through the contact form on www.50misconceptionsofsex.com and let me know if you are the exception to the rule and have not had any ejaculation for more than a month and the pain does not subside.

NO EJACULATION = BLUE BALLS

time they eventually evacuate after a long period of abstinence. I did... and it went away by itself. Of course, if pain persists, have your doctor check you for any medical condition like STDs. Just don't expect your regular doctor to have much experience with tantric practices or understanding why anyone would want to refrain.

What About Old Semen?

Another misconception (and fear) many men have is that the semen will stay inside the body and rot if they do not ejaculate. This is, medically speaking, *bullshit!* The body has the ability to break down and recycle un-used sperm.[2] For most men the body produced sperm before frequent ejaculation started. Instead of leaving the body, sperm was broken down and recycled. If you ejaculate frequently, then this recycling system goes into a sort of hibernation and becomes dormant. The re-awakening of your recycling system can be uncomfortable for a few days. It is almost always, just a one-off thing. In the meantime, here's some tips on how to relieve the discomfort:

Exercise

Cardiovascular exercise is great to burn up some of that extra energy. Although jumping rope may be the last thing you feel like doing, you can start with something less jarring. If you have the option, go for a swim, lift some weights or do some squats. Really, you can do any type of exercise that works the legs and lower body without too much bouncing.

Chill 'em

My doctor recommended taking the old boys for an ice cold dip. Here's a nice visual for you: I call it the *'frosty teabag'*. Dangle/dongle/dip your balls into a cup of cold water. (It makes for a hilarious spectator sport which I'm sure your friends would highly appreciate.)

A less spectacular variation is having a cold shower or taking a bag of frozen peas or ice in a damp hand towel that has been sitting in the freezer. (Hint: Place it in a Ziplock bag, so you don't have to peel it off your privates if it gets too cold). Remember, you won't have to do this for long,

---

2. https://www.thenakedscientists.com/articles/questions/
    what-happens-sperm-isnt-ejaculated

just until your body gets accustomed to your new sexual regime. A couple of minutes a day, for a day or so, is usually enough for the few guys who do feel any discomfort.

The Valsalva Maneuver

One last trick is the Valsalva Maneuver,[3] which you can simulate by picking up something heavy or bearing down as if you were on the toilet doing a #2. Although this technique is not recommended if you have a weak heart.[4] It helps relieve pressure long-term, by temporarily increasing blood pressure and thereby expanding the blood vessels.

Personally, I never use these techniques and just let the mild discomfort pass by itself, and it never returned... even after years of non-ejaculatory practice.

Photo credit: *Darko Djurin* (https://pixabay.com/users/derneuemann-6406309/), https://pixabay.com/photos/testicles-testicular-cancer-penis-2790218/

---

3. https://www.healthline.com/health/valsalva-maneuver
4. https://www.webmd.com/heart-disease/atrial-fibrillation/qa/what-are-the-risks-of-the-valsalva-maneuver

7

TOUCH THE CLITORIS FIRST

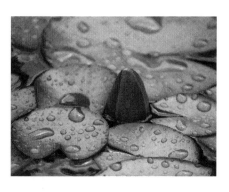

Reversing the Order

Let's talk a little more about the magic love-button, but this time more from the giver's perspective.

Hard to Resist the Clit

According to women who have practised sexual tantra for many years, touching the clitoris at the start of sex often makes a woman over-focus on it and get a little *'clit greedy'*. That old habit is often difficult to undo. The clitoral orgasm is the easiest orgasm for women to receive and it's also the least emotionally demanding. She doesn't need to surrender and can stay firmly in control.

From the perspective of the clit-educated man, the clitoris is the little button to show you care.[1] also an easy way to get some results and show you're not a *'dolt'*. So, ditching the clit from the sexual repertoire can create quite a lot of initial resistance from both sides. Long-term, let your brain do the neuroplasticity thing we mentioned in chapter 2, so you can trade up for better tantric orgasms.

---

1. https://www.menshealth.com/sex-women/a19531901/
    how-to-touch-her-clitoris-according-to-women/

A Better Way?

The main complaints I hear about someone being a bad lover is being too fast, being superficial, and too result-oriented.[2,3] See how direct clitoral stimulation can support that? I can understand clinging to it when there was no other alternative, but now that there are potentially more succulent items on the menu, it might be the time to revise that.[4]

If, as a man, you have maintained your sexual arousal without ejaculating for more than a couple of weeks, your body will become charged with non-greedy sexual energy with which you can do some really cool tantric shit. If you combine this energy with the skills outlined in this book, it will not be difficult at all to stand out from the crowd. Before long, you might even find that you are the one educating your female lover on the different orgasms available to women if they can abstain from clitoral orgasm.

Female Tops

There *is* a subset of the female population that *must* use their clitoris during sex, just as men require using their penis during sex.

I have a tantric lesbian friend who has always been a *'top'*. Her masturbation revolves around giving pleasure to the feminine with her imaginary penis. Even if she tries to be *'normal'* and fantasise about her vagina, her mind quickly switches back to her imaginary penis and her more habitual mode of being the active doer. Her physical masturbation routine involves *edging* whilst visualising she has a penis. (Remember that refers to very careful clitoral stimulation with fingers to 99% to the *'point of no return'* for long periods of time). Bottom line is, in her case, the pudendal nerve is her main sex organ, just like it is for men and their penises.[5]

In later chapters in this book, I talk about how female tops can use clitoral energy as a gift for others using sex toys, dildos and strap-ons. So, for these women, much of their energetic sexual practices will be closer to men's tantric practices. Having the same dominant position and nerves equals having the same energy flows, but as they have a woman's body,

2. https://www.psychologytoday.com/us/blog/the-power-pleasure/201209/orgasm-shouldnt-be-the-goal-sex-should-orgasm-be-avoided

3. https://www.huffpost.com/entry/how-to-radically-improve-_b_9223330

4. https://www.salon.com/2015/11/02/cervical_orgasm_partner/

5. https://www.sexcoaching.com/sexual-pleasure/edging-for-women/

they can take what works for them from both gender's practices.

Remember, this is just an experiment, and it is *your* body. In the end, researching and experimenting allows you to make a more informed decision about what is best for you. (Who said this book doesn't have its PC moments!)

Photo credit: *Jonny Lindner* (https://pixabay.com/users/comfreak-51581/), https://pixabay.com/photos/water-rose-lotus-lotus-blossom-354049/

8

MASTURBATION IS USELESS

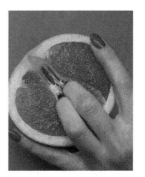

Indulge for a Good Purpose

Don't worry, there won't be any masturbation shaming going on in this book or warnings of hairy palms and such.[1] (Although, come to think of it, maybe little *Brillo Pad* action while you spank the monkey or pat the poodle could add a new spice in an otherwise routine solo endeavour?)

Seriously though, there are tantric ways to masturbate that can be done in a way that will actually make you a better lover. Let me paint you a picture of what masturbating in a tantric way can look like.

Love Shack

Tidy up your room, or at least throw the dirty laundry into the closet. Out of sight, out of mind! You want to make it look like a relaxed and beautiful space. If you live with other people, lock the door and maybe even put a notice up to indicate that you do not wish to be disturbed. Maybe, *'Spankin' it time'* is not the most appropriate sign if your grandmother likes to visit unannounced, but I'm sure you can work something out.

Set up your favourite sexy playlist. Turn off all the harsh lights in your room. If you have candles around, you can light a few (just to give it that tantric vibe), but any soft light source will do. Make sure you have some good oil or lubricant handy. Coconut oil and silicone lube are perfect for long-lasting slipperiness. Beware of water-based lube as it turns into glue after a few minutes in your hands whilst some women are allergic to silicone lubes in the vagina. Arrange the pillows and duvet in your bed and

---

1. https://www.medicalnewstoday.com/articles/320265.php#masturbation-side-effects

use a towel to protect your bedding.

Out with the Old, in with the New

By now, you probably have your go-to technique, and it may take some time to reprogram your body to become more sensitive to a way that leads you towards a deeper and healthier tantric sexuality.

Once you've got your sexy ambience sorted out, it's time for a little self-indulgence. Start by tossing the goal-oriented thoughts and behaviours out the window. This is not about some quick stress relief, but making you more present with what is actually happening in your body. Pay close attention, as this usually equates to becoming a better lover over time.

Focus on the actual sensations in your body rather than on any images in your head. Otherwise, you will reinforce the need to use your visual cortex to get horny, something you might want to avoid when you are with your partner.

Spread Your Legs

For the next step, open your body and don't contract or tighten any parts of it. By this, I mean *physically* open your legs while you masturbate, men included. Take a deep breath and relax your belly. If the body wants to make strange movements like jerking or twitching, then let that happen. Oftentimes, this is just your body's way of relaxing. Just keep breathing into it. The body knows how to open itself when your logical mind doesn't judge it as weird. Since your body has been running on about 5 to 10% of its sexual potential, it will need to open up internal channels to conduct a hornier energy through your body.

A Different Roadmap

You might be surprised by just how many other pleasurable spots there are for you to discover and enjoy.[2] Most female tantric practitioners avoid touching the clitoris and instead play with their breasts, stroke the labia, go inside the vagina, G-spot, cervix or anus. Create a new map of sensations. What does it feel like to touch different parts of your body when you are highly aroused? You might notice some places feel differently when your

---

2. https://www.healthline.com/health/healthy-sex/erogenous-zones#The-bottom-line

arousal and sensitivity levels are higher because of the tantric practice you are doing.

Men: Try not to use the regular *up-and-down-high-speed-jackhammer* movement with your hand. High-intensity stimulation desensitises your genitals over time and makes it more difficult to experience sexual arousal through light touch. The bigger the gap from your last ejaculation, the more intense a light touch will feel.

There is a technique that feels much closer to being inside a vagina. Turn your hand around so that your palm faces away from you and hold your penis in the palm of your hand. Mainly move the little finger and ring finger with a little movement of the palm. Your other hand can cup your balls or gently pull on your scrotum. Arch your back a little, as if you were lifting your tail. I know, it all sounds a little weird, but no one is looking, except that little critic in your head.

Another technique is to have the hand positioned in the same way, but squeezing your fingers together while you gently pull away from your body. With each stroke, it's like you're stretching and *'uncoiling'* the root of the penis. This movement is called *'jelqing'*, and some claim that, over time, it can unconstrict the base of the shaft that is pulled inside the perineum. Some go as far as saying that this technique can even give extra length to the part of the penis that is outside of the body.[3] I don't know how true this is, but in theory it makes sense, as you are not changing the actual length of the shaft, just moving it outwards.

Dildos and Butt-plugs, Good... Vibrators, Bad.

Dildos and butt-plugs can be useful for stimulating the g-spot, cervix and the prostate.[4] Vibrators are counterproductive in tantra because the aim is to regain virgin-like sensitivity, not lose it. Vibrators tend to desensitise genitals over time. If you've never used a vibrator before and you want to try them out, I can understand that, but prolonged use is not recommended. If you are familiar with vibrators, you might be familiar with *'vibrator creep'*. This refers to when women start off with the lowest setting and then, over time, need to buy the *Ultra Fat Max* that plugs into the wall

---

3. https://www.healthline.com/health/jelqing

4. https://www.bustle.com/p/what-are-the-benefits-of-butt-plugs-8-reasons-to-add-one-to-your-collection-18225995

socket.[5] Is this a good time to mention that building equipment companies rent out gasoline-powered industrial concrete vibrators? (I'm sure many of these jokes are working much better in my head than in yours.)

Heart Orgasms?

What I'm about to suggest may sound like some hippie bullshit, but some people report that long, tantric masturbation sessions can have a strong heart yoga kind of thing going on. I mean the *impersonal love and oneness with everything* gig. It seems to happen more by chance than as a volitional thing, but it does seem to occur with the right tantric practices.

Why Stay Horny?

The idea is to awaken your sexual energy and store it for more creative endeavours than the *crusty wank sock*. Perhaps you notice you think less about sex but feel a relaxed tingling in your body. Keeping that horny feeling alive in the body may make your creative thinking pop, especially when it comes to your highest potential for manifesting on Earth—your life's purpose.

Photo credit: *Ecosy* (https://www.shutterstock.com/g/ECOSY), https://www.shutterstock.com/image-photo/vagina-symbol-two-fingers-on-grapefruit-1022162836

5. https://www.bustle.com/articles/149233-only-orgasming-with-strong-vibrators-8-steps-to-regaining-sensitivity

9

CHILDBIRTH PAIN IS NATURAL

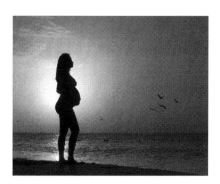

A New Way

Many of us probably have direct or indirect experience of traumatic childbirth, but does it really have to be like this? In my opinion, there is a lot tantra can do to improve current birthing practices. Does the pain (and indignity) of episiotomies, tearing of the perineum and caesarean sections seem a long way from natural? These regular child-birthing interventions can leave lasting sexual problems[1,2] Does it ever seem like a cruel trick of nature that potentially the most beautiful moment of life can also be one of the most painful and traumatising? Isn't it sad that the first sound a baby usually hears outside of the womb is the mother screaming in agony? Do I at least have your attention to hear about a natural pain-free tantric option to epidurals?[3]

Luckily there is one, and it's less expensive and simpler than many modern birthing methods. I'm talking about *'de-armouring'* the female reproductive organs and how to orgasm with the cervix and womb. We'll discuss these deeper orgasms in more detail later, but for now, let's focus on how to actually soften the vagina and cervix in preparation for a tantric birth.

---

1. https://www.today.com/health/
   episiotomies-tearing-after-childbirth-can-cause-lasting-painful-sex-t131701

2. https://parenting.nytimes.com/pregnancy/episiotomy

3. Cologne, Germany: Institute for Quality and Efficiency in Health Care (IQWiG); 2006-.
   Pregnancy and birth: Epidurals and painkillers for labor pain relief. 2006 Mar 3 [Updated
   2018 Mar 22]. Available from: https://www.ncbi.nlm.nih.gov/books/NBK279567/

De-armouring Explained

In a nutshell, de-armouring is the process of taking out numb and painful areas in the vagina using an internal pressure-point massage.[4] Some parts of the vagina, you can press hard without any pain. Other areas will have the woman weeping in pain from only moderate pressure.[5] Until the vagina is de-armoured, it can be rather tight and less elastic than might be naturally expected. Numbness or pain are sensations most often reported by the 2,500+ women who had their vaginas de-armoured at workshops, bodyworkers[6] or professionally trained tantric midwives.

Just to be clear, this process is not intended as therapy or medical healing. Women with medical issues such as severe vaginal tightness or dryness, vaginosis, cysts, diseases or other underlying medical conditions should see their doctor or professionally trained specialist before having de-armouring performed on them. Also do not perform or experiment with any de-armouring when the woman is pregnant (especially after week 37) as there is a real chance this practice may induce labour.

What Creates the Armouring?

Although I have never seen a scientific study done on this specific topic, there are several factors that seem to roughly correlate with the degree of armouring found in a woman's vagina and cervix:

- Chronic, high-stress
- Sexual abuse
- Shaming and sexual guilt
- Compromising and having sex out of obligation
- Frequent clitoral orgasms

The good news is that this hardening process can be reversed (with manageable levels of pain) in a relatively short period of time (50 minutes) and in most cases, it's a once-in-a-lifetime process.

---

4. https://www.health.harvard.edu/womens-health/
   pelvic-physical-therapy-another-potential-treatment-option

5. https://www.psychologytoday.com/us/blog/all-about-sex/201205/
   does-intercourse-hurt-guide-women-s-sexual-pain

6. www.thenewtantra.com

Vaginal De-Armouring 101

Here are the practical steps on how to de-armour a normally healthy vagina:

1. Lay down on your back and have a partner or close friend sit facing you, between your legs. Start with a brief massage on the belly and breasts to get connected. When you are relaxed enough, tell your partner you are ready to insert their fingers inside your vagina.

2. The de-armouring partner then investigates the walls of the vagina by pressing quite strongly with the fingers against the internal muscles. Once a painful point is reported by the woman, the partner should press firmly with constant pressure against the vaginal wall. Don't move or wiggle the fingers around on that spot, but rather hold that position for 2-3 minutes, until the pain subsides. The key here is for the woman not to tense up and fight against the pain. The *'tough-girl'* routine is counter-productive here. Instead, the woman should allow herself to become a vulnerable little girl. For women who spend a lot of time in their hard masculine side, this may be exactly where they do not want to go when feeling this pain.

3. If you're the one being de-armoured, express your uncomfortable feelings through verbal sounds such as moans and sobbing. You might go through a brief period of anger or screaming, but allow them to be gateways to even deeper vulnerability and sobbing. Think *'mommy, mommy'* and you will get the right idea. It's a surrendering experience rather than a *'tough it out'* experience. No vulnerability equals no de-armouring. Period.

4. The pain will usually go from *'intense'* to *'gentle discomfort'* within a couple of minutes on each spot. Once that part of the vagina stops hurting, move on to the next location and repeat the process. Cover all points—including the g-spot. The whole vagina usually takes about 35-40 minutes to de-armour and is usually completed in 1 session. However, it sometimes might require 2 or even 3 sessions.

After de-armouring, the vagina will often feel very different to the woman's touch; somehow softer, sensitive and more able to feel sexual energy during intercourse. The man can often sense a difference in how the vagina feels with his penis; more alive, energetic and horny, without the need for friction.

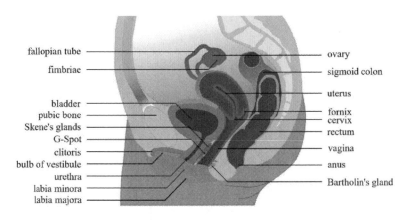

fallopian tube — ovary
fimbriae — sigmoid colon
— uterus
bladder —
pubic bone — fornix
Skene's glands — cervix
G-Spot — rectum
clitoris — vagina
bulb of vestibule —
urethra — anus
labia minora — Bartholin's gland
labia majora —

Now, the Cervix

If as a woman you've had sex that involved deep penetration, you may have had the unfortunate experience of feeling sharp pain when the penis hits a hardened cervix. What causes the pain is the same thing that causes pain during childbirth — lack of elasticity in the cervix.

Many women describe the pain of the penis hitting the cervix as feeling like a knife is cutting into them. Women seem to store stress and past trauma in this region more than anywhere else in the body. Even sexually experienced women will (unknowingly) control the depth and angle of penetration in order to keep the cervix away from the hard blows of a penis.[7] Doesn't this seem a little strange and unnatural when you think about it? Putting such a sensitive area right in the danger zone where it is going to get pumped and pummelled? Is it just a bad design flaw? It would seem so, unless there is a more evolved state of this delicate organ.

Here is how to de-armour the cervix with fingers. I will describe how to do it with the penis later in the book:

1. Once the vagina has been de-armoured, it will often be elastic enough to put several fingers inside, allowing the cervix to be gently squeezed (at first) between 2 fingers or, better yet, between a finger and thumb. Be prepared for a flood of overwhelming sensations,

---

7. https://www.bustle.com/p/
   how-much-pain-during-sex-is-normal-4-reasons-intercourse-may-be-hurting-12044331

emotions, unpleasant memories or possibly past trauma. Keep letting these emotions out through weeping or brief explosions of anger. This usually takes around 5-10 minutes.

2. The second phase of this process is signalled when the cervix pain reduces from *'knife-like'* to *'mildly unpleasant'*. At this point, the feeling can be transformed through intention into a sexual sensation.

3. Once there is virtually no pain, tapping and pressing on the cervix usually becomes progressively more arousing. Eventually, this alone can lead to a cervical orgasm that can last for several minutes.

4. Once the cervix has been de-armoured by fingers, short regular maintenance tune-ups are needed. This is better done with a penis or sitting on a dildo. I will described this step in further detail later in the book.

There are many benefits to a de-armoured vagina:

- Pain-free intercourse, even when the penis hits the cervix.
- Being able to feel the pleasure of frictionless sex without the need for movement.
- The resulting orgasms are longer, more intense and infinitely more satisfying than a clitoral orgasm.
- Women report that tantric orgasms do not deplete their energy in the same way as spasm orgasms do.
- A de-armoured vagina is necessary to experience the uterine womb orgasm, in which the entire area can erupt in convulsing orgasmic delight. (More on these types of orgasms in later chapters).
- The best news of all is that when a woman can regularly achieve the womb orgasm during sex, she will orgasm without pain during child-birth. (If you're into hidden symbols you might want to read the following footnote).[8]

---

8. As an interesting side-note, Genesis refers to women having pain during childbirth: Because Eve ate the *'forbidden fruit'* of the tree of knowledge... *'I [God] will intensify your labour pains; you will bear children with painful effort.'* This does not seem to have any relevance here unless we realise that the words *'know'* and *'sex'* are used interchangeably in the Bible. For example, Adam *'knew'* his wife Eve, and she conceived and bore a son, Cain. What could possibly be the forbidden fruit of a tree of sex? I'm not claiming there is any merit to this interpretation and subsequent coincidence between the Bible and tantric lore, but it does make an interesting story of the symbolism of the apple (the pudendal nerve *'shame'* orgasm, perhaps?) and the fall from innocence?

While this sounds totally fictitious to the uninitiated, have a read of this footnote[9] and perhaps watch some of the videos of women in rapture during child-birth.[10] Just google *'orgasmic birth'* for more information.[11] Here are also medically trained midwifes that have expanded their practice to include tantric knowledge and can perform de-armouring on the cervix before birth to assist with easier cervix dilation. And again, this should only be done by experienced and properly trained midwifes.

What a great way that must be to come into the world and start a new life, with your mother in rapture and pleasure instead of screaming in agony.

Photo credit: *Manuel Alejandro Leon* (https://pixabay.com/users/digitalmarketingagen cy-2670666/), https://pixabay.com/photos/beautiful-young-pregnant-woman-1434863/

Diagram credit: *Tsaitgaist https://commons.wikimedia.org/w/index.php?curid=8940986 UNDER the Creative Commons Attribution-Share Alike 3.0 Unported license*

9. Gaskin and others have noticed that woman in the throes of intense labour, and/or at the moment of birth, can look or behave as though they are experiencing orgasm (Gaskin 2003; Pascali-Bonaro 2007). Many women have described their child's birth in orgasmic language, or actually described having an orgasm at the moment of delivery (Baker 2001; Gaskin 2002, 2003; Shanley, 2008a, 2008b). Conducting her own casual survey, Gaskin found that 32 out of 151 interviewees reported having an orgasm at the moment of birth (Gaskin 2003). Similarities in the hormonal physiology of birth and orgasm, detailed below, underline this possibility. -'Essential Midwifery Practice: Intrapartum Care', Chapter 12, *'Sexuality in Labour and Birth: An Intimate Perspective'*, Sarah Buckley

10. https://www.youtube.com/watch?v=T0bsUUQfzCA

11. https://www.livescience.com/37039-orgasmic-birth-real.html

10

PERHAPS I'M GAY IF I ENJOY HER TOUCHING MY ASS

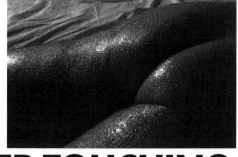

Anal De-Armouring

If as a man, you feel stigma of enjoying a woman touching your ass, there are plenty of reasons for that. Historically, in England and Wales, buggery was punishable by death.[1] In progressive Germany, fornication between men was not fully legalised until the late 1980s.[2] In Malaysia, sodomy is still punishable by imprisonment and a whipping.[3] Meanwhile, in the United States, sodomy laws were still valid until a 2003 Supreme Court case made fourteen states' laws unconstitutional.[4] Ten years later, American missionaries managed to convince the Ugandan government to put sodomy laws back on the books with a penalty of life imprisonment.[5] That seems rather a lot of interest in other peoples asses!

Does it ever strike you as strange why anyone would care, judge or take violent actions against what other consenting adults do in the privacy of

1. https://www.bl.uk/lgbtq-histories/articles/a-short-history-of-lgbt-rights-in-the-uk
2. https://news.stanford.edu/2018/12/29/east-germanys-lenient-laws-helped-unified-germany-become-gay-friendly/
3. https://www.theguardian.com/world/2012/jan/09/anwar-ibrahim-sodomy-dismissed-malaysian
4. https://journalofethics.ama-assn.org/article/decriminalization-sodomy-united-states/2014-11
5. https://harvardpolitics.com/covers/globalizing-hatred/

their own homes? You may well ask why many of the biggest advocates for action against gay men see themselves as religious?

Today's lobbyists often base their argument on homosexual behaviour being *'against nature'*.[6] However, why then do these same people usually only have a problem with gay men and not gay women? Even the most bro-like jocks, who make gay jokes and squirm at the thought of being considered homosexual, often fantasise about threesomes with attractive lesbian women. That is considered normal, but from a logical perspective it is still incoherent. Thus, it is unlikely that the non-baby-producing nature of homosexual sex is the real reason to outlaw this sexual act throughout the ages. Perhaps there is some other unconscious fear driving decisions to criminalising anal sex in such a wide variety of cultures.[7]

Getting Past Fear and Shame

As we discussed in the previous chapter of women storing stress in the cervix, similarly, we all seem to store fear and shame in the anus. Most people don't need an explanation of the meaning of the term *'pucker factor'*. If fear and shame is somehow emotionally stored in the anus, this would explain the fear of being forcefully sodomised without consent. Combine that with the gay-shame factor, and you have two very strong subconscious motives. In my youth, I clearly remember thinking I would kill myself if someone did such a thing to me. But logically, the fear of being anally raped can be addressed with general rape laws, so this doesn't explain the need for specific anti-sodomy laws between men. Perhaps the repulsion (and even the thought) of men enjoying anal play was abated by creating laws to hide it into the darkest most unseen corners. But perhaps this anal repulsion/fear could have been addressed in a more constructive way?[8]

Anal De-Armouring

Just as women can have their vagina and cervix de-armoured, both sexes can have their anuses de-armoured and stored fear and shame removed.

6. https://www.theguardian.com/world/2019/jun/01/texas-homophobic-laws-lgbt-unconstitutional

7. http://internap.hrw.org/features/features/lgbt_laws/

8. https://www.tandfonline.com/doi/abs/10.1080/15546128.2012.740951?scroll=top&needAccess=true&journalCode=wajs20

If you are a little squeamish about this subject, then you may want to skip over this chapter, otherwise, continue at your peril—as some people have an extreme reaction to this topic.[9] My advice is to try to adopt a doctor's demeanour on this subject. You can think of it as spiritual proctology or internal bodily yoga.

Looking from our new tantric perspective, when women give up the pleasure they experience from orgasming on the clit/pudendal nerve, they are able to experience a deeper pleasure through the pelvic, vagus and hypogastric nerves. Likewise, when tantric men choose to give up ejaculation, they open themselves up to the possibility of deeper stimulation through the hypogastric and pelvic nerves through the anus. Sorry guys, no vagus nerve orgasm for you because in men there is not a direct connection between the brain and the vagus nerve for some sexist biological reason!

Step by Step

Before we roll up our sleeves and jump in, let's start talking about how to deal with hygiene. An anal douche is a good idea. You can buy an anal douche or an enema at some pharmacies, good sex shops or online. An enema is a saline solution in a bottle with a slim tube that is inserted into the anus. An anal douche is a reusable bulb with a slim tip that is inserted into your butt (add some lube, or you'll be sorry). You can just use clean, potable water in the douche. The anal douche or enema will help you clear out most of the faeces from your rectum. You'll want to expel all of the water from your rectum. Repeat the process about 3 times or until the expelled water is clear.[10,11]

Use latex gloves. It's much more slippery, makes fingernails not so much of an issue, they're easier to clean up, and both parties can relax more. However, no matter how much cleaning you do, there's still the chance that someone might end up with a slightly poopy gloved finger. *Them's the breaks.* If your lover is willing, or better yet, if they're excited about getting to de-armour you, they probably won't care. Parents that love their babies seem to get over the whole shit issue remarkably quickly. It's a lot about

---

9. Branfman, J., Stiritz, S., & Anderson, E. (2018). Relaxing the straight male anus: Decreasing homohysteria around anal eroticism. Sexualities, 21(1–2), 109–127. https://doi.org/10.1177/1363460716678560

10. https://www.sfaf.org/collections/beta/anal-douching-safety-tips/

11. https://howtocleanyourass.wordpress.com/

the love factor.

Stored fear seems to accumulate in the muscles of the rectum and make it seem like it's closed for business, but gently dilating the *'puckered pooper'* is not a problem. We all do it at least once a day. Your partner will lube up their gloved hand, pour some more lube directly onto your ass and play with the entrance for a few minutes before you give the signal that you're ready for them to insert the finger... *slowly!*

The purpose is to help you learn to dilate your sphincter and eventually feel pleasure. Focus more on width than depth. Your anus is a muscle that is meant to spread open, just as you probably did this morning in your morning ablutions. You're asking your body to do the same thing but reversing the direction. With a little practice, insertion can even feel vastly more pleasant than elimination.

When strippers are first learning to dance, they are advised to dance slowly... and then go 50% of that speed... and then 50% of that speed again. Ask your partner to move *'stripper slow'* or *'Caribbean slow'*. And if that *still* feels too fast... Caribbean-stripper slow? (Finally, a nice visual!)

You can also play with the guy's penis at the same time as you are touching his ass. This seems to link the pleasurable horny sensations of the penis to the anus. Just be careful to stay below the *point of no return* as it can quickly get too horny when not in control in the same way as when on top.

One finger, two fingers, three, is all it takes. Just relax. As with yoga, you can't expect to do the *Wounded Peacock* on your first day. A full de-armouring luckily can take much more than one session as it's an acquired taste.

That Old Gay Question

Getting back to the title of this chapter, many men secretly fear that they will become gay if someone touches their ass and they start to enjoy it. On the contrary, many women testify that their men become better lovers (and thus more desirable) after they are de-armoured. Here are a few possible explanations:

- After de-armouring, the man is more relaxed in the base of the body and is now more sensitive and better able to feel and control the point of ejaculation. This increased sensitivity and awareness can mean that the man is able to have sex for longer periods and is better able to feel his partner's physical responses.

- The man is more likely to now be sympathetic and to have more empathy after having been in the position of receiving, and thus becomes better at reading and connecting with her more deeply. A man who has fully embraced the experience of having his own ass penetrated and who knows what it is like to be on the receiving end of a pleasurable anal experience is better equipped to orchestrate that event for someone else... just as a BDSM Dominatrix can improve her skills if she occasionally lives the experience as a submissive. So, my advice is to never let an ass virgin experiment on your ass. Better for them to learn on theirs, first!
- Men often report that they feel somehow recharged after receiving anal sex. Perhaps because anal de-armouring allows the man to relax and be served. I doubt people want to be in charge all of the time, it's exhausting! (We have a whole chapter coming up on this later).

So, if you want to experiment with a technique that might make you become a better lover and experience more pleasure yourself, perhaps give it a try. You probably won't lose any of your masculinity — in fact, the opposite is probably true. The main people who really get worked up and fixated on this topic are those who have some unrequited longing or repressed fear.

Methinks thou dost protest too much. —William Shakespeare.

Photo credit: *Klaus Hausmann* (https://pixabay.com/users/klaushausmann-1332067/), https://pixabay.com/photos/act-act-of-part-of-sex-sexy-man-3110289/

11

HETERO-SEXUALITY IS THE NATURAL WAY

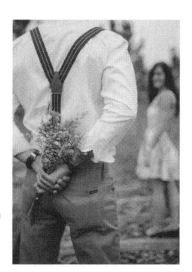

Define 'Natural'

Sexuality is a Spectrum

Dr Alfred Kinsey invented the Kinsey scale in the 1940s. This scale measured the degree of heterosexuality or homosexuality of an individual. The baseline of this scale is 0 if you're heterosexual, 6 if you're completely, flamingly G.A.Y.[1] Your female friend who likes to make out with other girls at the bar but then goes home with one of the guys watching is probably a 2 on this scale. Your gay friend who refers to women as *'fish'* or your lesbian friend who never lets her nails grow long are probably 6's. The point is that if we weren't so indoctrinated as to what is right and wrong, the vast majority of us might realise that we are on some kind of sliding scale. Due to shame, 100% heterosexual or homosexual is probably a lot more rare than publicly recognised.[2] Check for yourself. Didn't you also play doctors and nurses with boys *and* girls when you were a kid?

In itself, homosexuality is as limiting as heterosexuality: the ideal should be to be capable of loving a woman or a man; either, a human being, without feeling fear, restraint, or obligation. —Simone de Beauvoir

---

1. https://kinseyinstitute.org/research/publications/kinsey-scale.php
2. YouGov UK 2015 *"1 in 2 young people say they are not 100% heterosexual"* by Will Dahlgreen, https://yougov.co.uk/topics/lifestyle/articles-reports/2015/08/16/half-young-not-heterosexual

Since Kinsey's study, even more complex models of human sexuality have been developed. The Klein Sexual Orientation Grid, for instance, explores who you socialise with, who you fantasise about, and who you fall in love with.[3] This differs from Dr Kinsey's approach, which only looks at who you've had sex with and who you are aroused by.[4] So, if you identify as female, all of your friends are lesbians, and you fantasise about sex with women but you mostly end up with men, you might only be a 1 on the Kinsey Scale (due to your actions), but with the Klein Sexual Orientation Grid, you might be more accurately represented by capturing more nuances of your sexuality. Both of these models lack the ability to describe the sexual attraction to people whose gender is not easily defined as male or female. (More on this in the next chapter.)

Think about what kind of people you like. Do you feel comfortable around masculine men or men who are softer and dress more feminine — the metrosexual? Some bisexuals prefer to only date other bisexuals. Some non-binary people prefer to date other non-binary people. In a gender-fluid world, there are a lot of new possibilities for the brave and open-minded.

The take-home consideration is that it may be more unusual than commonly accepted to be attracted to a narrow gender band. As a gender-fluid person myself, I am continually surprised by the high percentage of straight men (and women), that are attracted to me. It's quite frustrating that the silent majority is afraid of cultural shaming and being socially outcast if they express openly their appreciation of anything that does not fit the sexual norm.[5] Only by living as a gender-fluid person does one get to experience first-hand the large percentage of people silently living in their silo of sexual shame.

Think about the range of people you have been attracted to in the past and, in particular, think about the people who you are privately attracted to but are ashamed for your friends to find out about. Labels make it even harder to admit when your interests don't align with your chosen public persona.[6] If you identify as a straight man, but you are attracted to feminine cross-dressers, it doesn't mean you have to lose your straight-man

3. http://www.americaninstituteofbisexuality.org/thekleingrid

4. http://www.lgbtdata.com/kinsey-scale.html

5. https://janetmock.com/2013/09/12/men-who-date-attracted-to-trans-women-stigma/

6. https://www.psychologytoday.com/us/blog/finally-out/201107/the-messy-realities-bisexuality

accolade. It might actually mean that you are confident enough in your heterosexuality that you realise that you are attracted to the feminine form, irrespective of genitalia. What man doesn't love his own dick? In fact, I find the men who are most confident in their heterosexuality and simply love the feminine form are the ones who will take me out to a nice restaurant and don't care what others think.

Can't We All Just Get Along?

How certain are we that our sexual preference really comes from a free-thinking space? That we have not been unknowingly conditioned by society to accept heterosexuality as the norm? I certainly was.

One interesting thing that I have observed in the de-conditioning of people's sexuality is that most people become 'hetero-flexible' if they deeply voyage into the courageous zone of self-exploration. Hetero-flexibility refers to people whose primary attraction is to the opposite sex, but have transcended their sexual fear or repulsion of the same sex. Interestingly, gay men and women often become 'homo-flexible' as they develop and become more de-conditioned.

It is one thing to be attracted to persons of a specific gender, but another thing to be repulsed by a specific gender. Repulsion is usually connected to past trauma or conditioning. It's often quite obvious when you hear gay men talking about how gross women's vaginas are or hardcore dykes talking about penises being repulsive, as there is surely nothing inherently gross about either sex's genitals... just a past story associated with it.

Many gay men do seem to love boobs though, so maybe breasts are the gateway to homo-flexibility?[7] Lesbians sometimes love the shape of a cock. OK. There! I've said it! They're usually not so excited about dating a man with a cock, but aren't most lesbian sex toys in the shape of a penis? You might be surprised by how often I've been propositioned by women who identify as lesbian. They seem to be open to me as long as I press the female visuals button, and a penis under the dress can sometimes be seen as a bonus rather than a liability, at least for the most liberal.

---

7. https://www.outfrontmagazine.com/trending/culture/stuff-gay-people-like-breasts/

Playing Doctors and Nurses

Whilst hetero-flexibility may not come as a shock to most women, the average man may need a little more of a sexual segue. (Not that I am under the delusion that an average man would have read this far into this rather alternative book!) Let's investigate your own childhood for any possible signs of sexual preference limiting through sexual-conditioning.

Between the ages of 3 and 6, it is normal for children to engage in spontaneous, innocent, consensual sexual play with their friends of a similar age.[8] When you were a child, did you play sexual games? If you are indeed in the majority that did, were you limited to only the opposite sex, or did you play with both sexes? Of the thousands of adults whom I've asked this question, about 80% of people say they were sexually playful as a child. Of those naughty kids, 95% say that they played with *both* genders. It seems from those statistics that hetero-flexibility may be a naturally occurring interest and curiosity that later gets conditioned through upbringing to stick to the straight and narrow.

How do you know you are a 0 on the Kinsey scale and 100% straight? Disinterest... not repulsion. The opposite of interest is *disinterest*. According to sexologists and sex therapists, repulsion is usually a sign of repressed interest.

Homophobia is more prevalent in people who have an unacknowledged attraction to the same sex and who grew up with authoritarian parents who openly criticised LGBT people and culture. Individuals who identify as straight but in psychological tests show a strong attraction to the same sex may be threatened by gays and lesbians because homosexuals remind them of similar tendencies within themselves. —Dr Netta Weinstein, from the University of Essex.[9]

I am in no way saying that people's attractions need to be changed... or that there is any merit being one way or another. I am merely observing that when people engage in sexual de-conditioning, they tend to become more sexually open, and may even have sexual contact with people they formerly avoided. Revulsion may be a coping mechanism for preventing being ostracised or harmed by those who judge us or an early survival

8. https://www.nctsn.org/sites/default/files/resources/sexual_development_and_behavior_in_children.pdf

9. http://www.revelandriot.com/study-homophobia-is-often-a-sign-of-latent-homosexuality-86569/

strategy to gain appreciation from our caregivers.

Cultural Conditioning

Have you ever been bullied in the schoolyard as a *'poofter'*, gay or queer? These are generally slurs aimed at boys. Men are generally more strongly pressured to be straight than women.[10] Lesbian sex is seen as hot by most people, and the vast majority of the women I have surveyed usually masturbate to girl-on-girl sex. In fact, girl-on-girl is the #1 searched for porn category by women.[11] Women naturally seem to have a bisexual side that hasn't been conditioned out of them through bullying and other forms of social pressure.[12] Thus, there does not seem to be as much shame about women being hetero-flexible as there is with men.

In contrast, even men who played doctor with other boys during childhood, usually convert exclusively to heterosexuality if someone shamed them. Men sometimes bury those guilty childhood memories deep into the forgotten past. I'm not saying that most of us would fall in love with the same sex if we were totally de-conditioned, but consider that when people lose their memories through mental disabilities, they often can't remember their sexual preference.[13]

The Chemistry of Sexuality

There have been scientific experiments indicating that changing hormones and neurotransmitters in rats can change their sexual preference. Researchers from the *Universidad Veracruzana*, Mexico, have been able to show that conditioned homosexual preference in male rats can be induced by oxytocin and the psychoactive drug *quinpirole*, which is known to have the same effect on the brain as the neurotransmitter dopamine.[14]

---

10. https://www.pewsocialtrends.org/2013/06/13/chapter-2-social-acceptance/

11. https://www.psychologytoday.com/us/blog/all-about-sex/201803/
surprising-new-data-the-world-s-most-popular-porn-site

12. Lisa M. Diamond PhD (2007) The Evolution of Plasticity in Female-Female Desire, Journal of Psychology & Human Sexuality, 18:4, 245-274, DOI: 10.1300/J056v18n04_01

13. Miller BL, Cummings JL, McIntyre H, Ebers G, Grode M. Hypersexuality or altered sexual preference following brain injury. J Neurol Neurosurg Psychiatry. 1986;49(8):867–873. doi:10.1136/jnnp.49.8.867

14. http://www.iflscience.com/brain/
sexual-preference-rats-influenced-oxytocin-and-dopamine/

HETEROSEXUALITY IS THE NATURAL WAY

How sure is the average person that their sexual preference would not change if given the right cocktail of drugs? I also wonder how many men would not only masturbate but actually perform *fellatio* on themselves if they were flexible enough to do so. Most men I ask this hypothetical question often admit a timid, *'yes'*. Maybe it is not actually the penis that straight men are not attracted to, but the male body. What if transsexuals were thought of as normal, or even an honoured part of society? I guess many heterosexual men might still have sex with Angelina Jolie if she had a penis. Hmmmm, now there is an interesting thought... (No disrespect intended to Angie. How can anyone hate that incredibly talented, sexually relaxed, altruistic, brave and highly interesting woman? Well I guess that's precisely why according to Rene Girard's *Mimetic Desire Theory*.)[15]

Finally, if bisexuality is a unique result of human neuroticism, why then is bisexuality so regularly observed and well documented in the animal kingdom?[16]

My goal in sharing this information is not to convert anyone, (except maybe George Clooney and Denzel Washington :p), but if you think that you are the only one with weird private fantasies involving people who are not, strictly speaking, the opposite gender, you might not want to judge yourself quite so quickly. I certainly won't.

Photo credit: *Alice Bitencourt* (https://pixabay.com/users/aliceabc0-1104247/), https://pixabay.com/photos/nature-love-couple-in-love-grooms-1790142/

---

15. https://woodybelangia.com/what-is-mimetic-theory/
16. https://en.wikipedia.org/wiki/Homosexual_behavior_in_animals

12
MEN ARE
MASCULINE

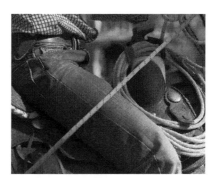

Beyond
Stereotypes

Women sometimes say that they want their partner to *'be a man'* or to be *'more masculine.'* What do they mean by this, exactly?

For a full answer to this question, I would like to point you in the direction of David Deida. He devoted an entire book on this subject, titled *'The way of the superior man'*. He does more justice to this subject than I possibly can in one chapter, so I will only cover a few additional points that I can add.[1]

What this book specialises in is the alternative and newer aspects of practical modern tantra and how it is evolving in recent times. One recent trend is the interest in gender-fluidity in the fashion industry which is often at the forefront of more widely accepted trends. I also use the terms *masculine* and *feminine* in the same way that Deida does. Both biological men and women contain feminine and masculine qualities within themselves in different ratios. Traditionally, the average woman has a bigger feminine side than masculine and vice-versa for men. There is also a smaller minority of men and women where these ratios are reversed, but there is no implication that men should be masculine or women should be feminine. I will be using the terms *masculine* and *feminine* in a non-gender way throughout this book.

---

1. https://deida.info/the-way-of-the-superior-man/

The Gender Spectrum

Traditionally certain cultures have recognised a third gender.[2] Different countries have different names and different social roles for gender fluid people. For example, eunuchs are castrated men who guard women's quarters.[3] There are the *Fa'afafine* from Samoa, who are born male but engage in traditional women's work and sometimes dress and behave like women as well.[4] *Kathoeys* in Thailand are an integral part of Thai culture, whilst the *Albanian Sworn Virgins* are women that dress and live as men.[5]

More recently in the West you'll see a growing number of people whose gender can't be so easily determined.[6] In cities like London, New York, Amsterdam and San Francisco, you'll see more varieties of gender expression every year.

Gender seems to become a more fluid spectrum than a fixed pigeon-hole. To represent this, Liat Wexler developed the *Universe Model of Gender* to represent specific types of people loosely clustered together in a gender universe, rather than being limited to anatomical gender.[7] The lines are progressively blurring.

How to Define Gender

There are scientific markers of gender called chromosomes. Usually, women have XX and men have XY, but there are a lot of variations and there are also humans whose genetic sex and genitalia do not match.[8,9]

Hormones are another way of defining gender but recently in the news, there has been a furore in sports over women who have naturally occurring

2. http://www.pbs.org/independentlens/content/two-spirits_map-html/
3. https://www.britannica.com/topic/eunuch
4. https://www.bbc.com/news/world-asia-37227803
5. https://video.nationalgeographic.com/video/00000144-0a35-d3cb-a96c-7b3d87520000
6. https://www.cnn.com/2018/02/06/health/teens-gender-nonconforming-study-trnd/index.html
7. http://wiki.preventconnect.org/wp-content/uploads/2018/08/Universe-Model-of-Gender-2015.pdf
8. https://www.livescience.com/27248-chromosomes.html
9. https://www.mayoclinic.org/diseases-conditions/ambiguous-genitalia/symptoms-causes/syc-20369273

high levels of testosterone.[10] This is only one of the many ways in which nature defies the clear-cut cultural boundaries between male and female, confounding scientists and legislators alike.[11] At what point does a girl's testosterone level become too high for a girl to be allowed to compete with other girls? At what point does that testosterone level push her into a category to more fairly compete with men than women? But outside of sports do we really need to define people into one gender pigeon hole or other?

Both is Better

Although it may sound counter-intuitive, men can actually become more masculine by consciously spending some time in their feminine side. I guess most of us can logically understand that being hyper-masculine 24/7 would lead to burnout. Thus, relaxing into the feminine makes sense as a way to bounce back and feel excited about being in charge again. Even small things like getting a massage, a spa manicure, nature walks or dancing are ways to get in touch with the feminine side. In fact playing around with gender roles is not a new idea and is in fact a key aspect of tantra. For example, Buddhist tantric practitioners often visualise themselves as deities of opposite gender.

One measure of personal growth could be to become better in the masculine, feminine or preferably both sides. I would suggest you might want to avoid the common mistake of not being particularly good at either.

The main reason why I love being able to live out both genders is that I have more opportunities to practise living two lives and work at being stronger in both. As the *Kinky Boots* song proclaims *'The world seemed brighter, 6 inches off the ground.'* Practising in an arena that was traditionally off limits to your native gender can be quite a transformative experience, and often gives a subjective appreciation for the hard fought opportunity to explore roles that others may take for granted. As evidenced by *Ru Paul's Drag Race*, some of the most creative make-up and costume designs are done by gender fluid people, and may explain why there is often a talented metrosexual guy enthusiastically working in makeup shops like MAC.

---

10. https://www.sciencedaily.com/releases/2019/02/190212160030.htm
11. https://www.npr.org/2019/05/31/728400819/i-am-a-woman-track-star-caster-semenya-continues-her-fight-to-compete-as-a-femal

People often find it unusual how masculine I am when I am in guy mode. I am certainly more masculine than I was before I started cross-dressing. One of my theories on this subject is that perhaps an unmet feminine longing in men may weaken the masculine. Perhaps fully living out the feminine side for a while, later catapults one back into the masculine with renewed enthusiasm and vigour.

Understanding Other

I'm not deluded into thinking that putting on a dress makes me a woman but, what I did notice was that my thoughts changed quite dramatically when I switched from being in my masculine mode to my feminine mode. Furthermore, I was able to study my feminine mind from the contrast of my internal, masculine, detached perspective.

Most of what I learned about feminine longing was not learned through studying, but by becoming gender-fluid. Learning how to direct a woman into her feminine longing to surrender became simply obvious after being in that position myself. If a picture paints a thousand words, then living it must be closer to a million.

Photo credit: *Patrick Gantz* (https://pixabay.com/users/caropat-3683851/), https://pixabay.com/photos/horse-saddle-jumper-lasso-cowboy-1955278/

13

WOMEN ARE FEMININE

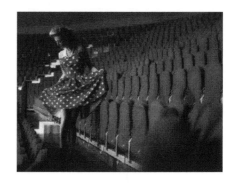

Feminine is Energy

Traditionally, one way to distinguish the masculine practices from feminine practices is the *transformational* aspects of tantra. Let me explain. Instead of the traditional masculine spiritual practices of *piercing through* situations to emptiness, the hardship of renunciation or even avoiding temptations and strong emotions in provocative situations to cultivate equanimity (sutra), the traditional feminine or tantric path is to fully indulge and immerse yourself in increasingly intense situations and *transform* darkness into light (whilst not getting lost in the process). For those interested in a more in-depth knowledge on this subject I highly recommend the brilliant summary by David Chapman.[1]

As we mentioned in the last chapter, my use of masculine and feminine is gender neutral, as it is simply good practice for all of us to more deeply embody both our masculine and feminine qualities to expand our human capacities.[2] In this chapter we will focus on expanding the feminine spectrum and see how it relates to sexual attraction and polarity.

Women usually have no shame in activating their masculine qualities in the workplace and can obviously do just as good a job as men can. Studies show men and women have the same level of intelligence,[3] the challenge

1. https://vividness.live/2013/10/23/sutra-vs-tantra/

2. https://www.inc.com/jessica-stillman/want-to-learn-faster-make-your-life-more-unpredictable.html

3. https://www.apa.org/action/resources/research-in-action/share

is that even in the home, it is often the woman who directs the family and is activating her masculine there as well, which can lead to issues when she becomes tired of always being in the draining masculine role.[4]

Polarity Problems

After a long day in the office handling paperwork, dealing with clients and bosses and dodging the office creep, she fights her way home through traffic or on public transportation… to find there's more to handle at home to keep the house organised and running.[5] Does the laundry need to be done or the dishwasher run? Maybe she still needs to make sure that the family is fed.[6] If she never gets to wind down, she may just continue to use her masculine mode to handle everything, including her male partner. This is the most common polarity-killing mistake in relationships. A woman might be comfortable kicking butt with the best of men at work, but she will probably need the exact opposite skills if she wants to take a more feminine role with her masculine partner.[7]

Opposites attract. So what happens if both partners are trying to direct with their masculine, or they are both passively waiting in their feminine for the other to take direction? It's called *lack of polarity*. There isn't a problem with lack of polarity *if* you are both not interested in being sexually attracted to each other.[8] But, what if you *are* interested, and you can't get the embers to glow anymore? In that case, understanding polarity is key. Otherwise, you'll be flogging a dead horse and not understanding why old Betsy ain't winning at Ascot.

Trying to get a dormant sex life restarted through complaining is the most common mistake. Complaining is a sure-fire method to emancipate and kill attraction. If you don't believe me, try this little experiment with the hubby and measure the results in *sack shrinkage*. *'Why can't you just be more of a man!'* This is certainly one way to keep his balls in your pocket…

---

4. https://www.psychologytoday.com/us/blog/science-practice/201908/tired-doing-the-invisible-work-in-your-family

5. https://www.huffpost.com/entry/7-reasons-your-wife-is-st_b_6621940

6. https://www.nytimes.com/2018/11/14/smarter-living/stress-gap-women-men.html

7. https://www.insider.com/modern-dating-coach-explains-why-high-achieving-women-struggle-to-find-love-2019-3

8. https://www.huffpost.com/entry/power-dynamics-in-sexual-_b_9843280

and foster temporary erectile dysfunction... which may not exactly be the result you were hoping for!

So, let's look at the simple mechanics of restoring polarity. Someone following and someone leading is the simplest way. We will go into this and other solutions in much greater detail in the next chapter, but the long-term (and more difficult) solution is for both partners to practise being either more masculine or more feminine at any given moment. We will discuss cultivating masculinity in more detail in chapter 40, so this chapter will concentrate on how to create polarity through feminine practices.

In a traditional heterosexual relationship, if the man loses attraction to his woman, one possible reason is that he may be suffering from a restrict-ed diet of all the possible feminine energies that she could potentially be offering him. He may be saturated with one or two flavours she habitually presents (such as the mother, the nurturer or the wise woman), but is starving for other flavours. Only supplying one or two of these flavours is the equivalent of restricting a woman to wearing only one or two different colours, shoes or dresses for a year. I think I would have an arrhythmic myocardial infarction if that was forced on me. (I am always looking for a situation to use that big fancy medical term for heart attack, because I secretly wanted to be a doctor when I was a kid but alas, wasn't smart enough.)

Not practising to broadening the feminine spectrum to include as many flavours as possible, the variety of offerings will become limited and some-what monotonous. But why would anyone limit their offering to someone they love?

Resistance

Perhaps the woman may long to get out of her masculine *'thinking head'* mode and surrender into her feminine body by using tools like singing, dancing or running a bubble bath, but she may also feel (from her stressed masculine side), that these are frivolous time-wasting activities that she doesn't have time for. They become low-priority when compared to screaming kids, which is both understandable and a shame if it takes its toll on her *joie de vivre* and the relationship.

There's also a vulnerability that comes with the softer feminine side, so always operating in tough masculine mode can be an emotional safe haven. After showing the world her invulnerable face at work all day, it can be difficult for a woman to take off the armour and open herself up to connect with the ones she loves. She may feel resentful about having to take on the lion's share of the household chores, and resentment can easily turn into a hard, impenetrable Kevlar shell.[9] Keeping it all together might signal to her partner that she doesn't need help, whereas breaking down and showing him how it feels to constantly force her feminine body to activate its masculinity might create a much needed vacuum for him to step-up and take back the reins.

Energy Shame

So what is the answer? If you want to practise expanding your female repertoire, see how many different types of feminine energy you can command and bring to bear at will. Maybe you are comfortable in certain flavours of the feminine but resist others. Nurturing-mother-mode may be a crowd-pleaser with kids, relatives and girlfriends, but not a big boner inducer for hubby.[10]

It's not that it's physically impossible for women to access different flavours of the feminine, but that there is a conditioned resistance that makes them think that certain areas of the feminine spectrum are wrong or demeaning. One good practice is the slow but steadily incremental over-coming of societal conditioning and learning to embody a wider spectrum at will. It's like having a shelf full of different herbs and spices and being able to pull out whatever condiment is needed to lift a bland beef stew into a tasty vindaloo.

Of course, many people like to pretend that this is not the case, as we should simply *'love each other exactly as we are'*. As I often say, *'if you think you are perfect the way you are, you probably have low standards'*. The danger with pretending is that a silently starving guy may often start looking outside of the relationship to get the flavours he desires when he could be receiving it in a less destructive way at home.

Although this might be an uncomfortable truth, us feminine beings have the opportunity to broaden our practice by embodying a whole spectrum of feminine energies and providing the most desired ones to our partners

9. https://www.theatlantic.com/sexes/archive/2013/03/the-difference-between-a-happy-marriage-and-miserable-one-chores/273615/

10. https://www.psychologytoday.com/us/blog/in-the-name-love/201609/women-s-right-say-yes-sexuality

when they need it. This will create less chance for unfulfilled longings to sabotage the relationship. Learning how to move with ease between different feminine archetypes means that you have greater feminine embodiment abilities and thus a greater capacity to attract a deeper man.

This is a very short introductory chapter on this topic, and I would like to refer you whole-heartedly to a much fuller explanation on this topic in the book *'Dear Lover'* by David Deida.[11]

Photo credit: *Alexandr Ivanov* (https://pixabay.com/users/ivanovgood-1982503/), https://pixabay.com/photos/pin-up-girl-pin-up-dress-red-arena-1595489/

---

11. https://deida.info/read/dear-lover-online/

14

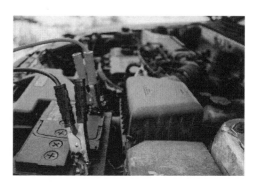

SEX REQUIRES EFFORT

The Secret of Effortless Sexual Energy

Let's look at the solution to the problem of lack of sexual energy in a relationship. The most common feedback from sexologists and marriage guidance counsellors is to spice things up with novelty and variety.[1] This can take several forms, like paying more attention to your appearance, role playing sexy scenarios, buying lingerie or a new sex toy.[2] This type of advice seems rather superficial and its results usually have more of a temporary Band-Aid-like effect than a permanent sea-level shift.

It's a sensitive and emotionally charged subject and thus it is often easier to see the situation more clearly by looking at others. Let's take the example of 'lesbian bed death'.[3] This is when a lesbian couple stops having sex and just lives their relationship as celibate sisters. While love and friendship are there, the fire is gone. The cause might be that the one who used to be the initiator and took on more of the masculine role got tired. Perhaps she has taken on more responsibility at work and now has to spend more time in her masculine side during the day. It's possible that she still enjoys taking

1. https://www.huffpost.com/entry/sexless-marriage-advice-therapists_n_5a7348bde4b09 05433b2102f

2. https://www.oprahmag.com/life/relationships-love/a28427355/ how-to-spice-up-sex-life-tips/

3. https://www.lesbiannews.com/the-truth-and-myth-of-the-lesbian-bed-death/

on the masculine role but she also needs some downtime in her feminine, so she can recover and feel excited again about tapping into her masculine essence to initiate sex with her partner with a more feminine essence. The same scenario can obviously apply to a heterosexual relationship.[4] The vast majority of long-term marriages are often sexless due to this same dynamic. Both people are too tired to initiate a roll in the proverbial hay.[5]

If this describes you and your relationship, you may want to see what happens if you nurture your partner who used to initiate sex but seems to have lost interest. What happens if you put them in a bubble bath and wash their hair or rub their feet? Any kind of sweet nurturing activity that allows them to relax in the feminine surrendering mode could provide enough recuperation to allow the pendulum to swing back towards the initiating masculine.

A lot of high-powered, successful men secretly live out (or crave) being in their surrendering and submissive side. Many women are able to make a living as dominatrixes because successful and powerful men are willing to drop considerable amounts of cash to relax and submit. A domination session might be the only time when he doesn't need to be *in charge*, and thus will be able to *recharge* his draining *being on top of things* side. The technique of adopting the traditionally feminine traits of surrender somehow seems to hit a reset button and acts as the highest-speed form of recharging.

Switching Roles

To create attraction, simply designate one person as the leader and the other as the follower. The difficulty, however, is if neither wants to lead. When both are tired, it can be difficult to conjure up enough energy to nurture the other and get the party started. This is a scenario in which there may be unexplored potential for the woman to tap into her masculine sexual side. Here's a sexperiment you can try the next time he doesn't seem interested in you, or when you are both simply too exhausted to take the initiative.

Let's say you are a regular married couple with kids and little sex. You

---

4. http://www.pattigeier.com/thetruthaboutlesbianbeddeath.py
5. https://www.everydayhealth.com/sexual-health-pictures/reasons-youre-too-tired-for-sex.aspx

are open to the idea to have sex with each other, but you both are hoping for the other to take the lead. There is a little trick you can do that I originally learnt from the Deida books. It may seem counterintuitive, but one of the most effective ways out of this gridlock is for the woman to use her remaining masculine energy in a way that is primarily fun for her (and him as a by-product). This means the woman initiating. Wait, wait! Before you roll your eyes at sweet little me, I *do* realise that in a long-term relationship, family and a regular busy schedule may leave you feeling constantly tired, but hear me out... there is a good ROI here (return on investment) for any energy you invest.

Here's how it works. Offer to play a sex game with him for 20 minutes. In this game, the woman (in this example), is in charge and gets to do whatever she wants with him. If he agrees (most likely, he'll do it, if he doesn't have to initiate anything) you get to explore what would be fun for you to do. Think along the line of using him (in a nice way) as your personal sex toy. You can even start by thinking out loud, suggest this or that, and if either of you particularly likes an idea, then you can move to the next stage of actually doing it. In this way, you can propose even the weirdest creative ideas without the risk of being rejected. You might be surprised how much a man will let you do to him, as long as he doesn't have to make any decisions. We'll get to some examples in a minute, but let's finish the theory first.

Usually, a man only needs to be in the sexual feminine for a relatively short period of time before his batteries become fully charged. The reason is that most men have a smaller feminine side and thus a smaller feminine need and it takes less time to recharge them. This is why, in the average hetero couple, it works better to recharge the man's batteries first, as hers will take a lot longer to recharge, as she will typically have a deeper longing to surrender in her true feminine core.

There will be little doubt as to when his feminine battery is full because he will suddenly become impatient to switch from submissive to dominant and want to be in the driver's seat again. This is quite different from being pressured by *'Why can't you be more masculine and just take me!'*

The ROI that I referred to earlier is that if he is something like the average man with 25% feminine and 75% masculine, his inherent capacity to be in his masculine and lead is 3 times greater... How much he will actually be able to manifest this capacity will depend on his level of practice.

How to Lead?

All right. How to actually get it all started? Besides tiredness, most women also report an initial emotional resistance to taking the lead. Oftentimes, it seems to come from the feeling of being unsure what to do. Don't sweat it. It will come back to you. Just let yourself rediscover the playful girl inside. Your infinitely creative side might be just under the surface, waiting for permission. We all instinctively knew how to play when we were children, even though we had less cognitive abilities. The secret is to not take it too seriously. Laughter can be a great aphrodisiac.[6] Err on the side of wild and crazy, and experiment with as many scenarios as cross your mind. Almost anything is better than nothing, and in trying different things, you might learn new things about your partner, even after years of knowing them. Quite quickly, most women usually find that they do have a playful sexually-dominant streak in them.

You don't have to be an expert at leading and finding the perfect things to do. Just the fact that he doesn't have to make any decisions can be a blissful break from the masculine pressure to perform. For a man, there can be an immense pleasure just in enjoying watching your sexual pleasure and surrendering to your desires, especially if he has been the one traditionally on top, in your relationship.

Here's another example of recharging sexual batteries in reverse order to the previous example to give you some more ideas:

I am exhausted. I feel like I've run a marathon. Over the last hour, I have completely depleted my sexual energy battery pack. I have been the one doing most of the physical exercise as well as doing the masculine directing and guiding. I've got nothing left to give. I desperately need some recharging.

Luckily, she is full of energy and has spent most of the time on her back. Feminine is another name for being the receiver, the one surrendering. It is now time to balance the equation. I need to go into my feminine, receptive side. Time for her to take charge. She has found her masculine sexual hunger and enjoys playing with me and watching me surrender. She loves getting to play with me as her sex toy. I feel a flush of energy enter my body just at the prospect of being used for a while. It feels so great not having to be in charge all of the time, fun to not know what is going to happen next and I

---

6. https://www.psychologytoday.com/us/blog/emotional-fitness/201905/
   the-two-sides-humor-in-relationships

love seeing her authentically enjoy herself.

For a minute, I forget my role. 'I'm ready... but could you please close the window first babe?' She doesn't miss a beat...

'Ah! Excuse me? Who's directing whom here, my dear? Do you want to be in charge again?'

'No, no! Sorry...!'

'Then, simply express your current status and let me decide what should be done about it.'

'OK... Let me rephrase that... I'm a little cold.'

'Much better... Let me close the window for you.'

I love this game. I don't have to decide shit... but old habits die hard.

Out comes the oil and she proceeds to turn me into an organic slippery-dip. I hope these aren't our best sheets.

Teaching Without Words

There is another hidden benefit for you to sometimes lead, Miss. This is your chance to teach him first-hand what you long for, without having to use words.

Do you long to be lovingly and skilfully manhandled? If so, show him exactly how you would like it done to you. Lean over him, cradle his neck in the crook of your elbow and position him where you want him on the bed. Do you want him to pin you down and kiss your neck? Then, show him that. Do you like to be *playfully* gagged? Maybe take your G-string off and stuff it in his mouth, whispering in his ear that he is yours until you're finished with him. Show him some of the things you would like him to do. Maybe not his boxers in your mouth, but you get the general gist of things, right?

As you physically dominate him, pay close attention to his bodily responses so you can see what works without needing words. This is, perhaps, the single greatest skill to learn for both partners: how to lead by following responses. By showing, you don't have to tell him what he could do better. Men usually have very fragile sexual egos, and they can shut down or rebel if you tell them directly what they are doing wrong. Same goes with making too many requests while having sex. It is much better to give him the direct experience of being in the feminine position. He then won't need to bumble around and guess so much about how to fulfil your feminine longings because he has been sexually schooled by you.

> *She seems to know exactly what I need to open and surrender... as if it were second nature to her. Well, I guess it is, as she has spent her entire adult sexual life in the feminine position... and probably much of that wishing what I could have done better. Now she gets her chance to show me how it's done.*

Clothing

Clothing is one of the easiest and most fun ways to switch roles. You might remember how much fun it was to play dress-up when you were young. It might be enjoyable for you to see him a little more vulnerable (and out of his comfort zone), dressed very differently. Think of it as a grown-up, dress-up time. It might be more interesting than Netflix tonight.

When I first started leading tantra workshops, I suggested that men should not be ashamed of experimenting with their feminine side... and that might also include clothing. I assumed that very few would be willing to experiment or, even less, to enjoy cross-dressing. I assumed it was just my weird side projected onto others. Much to my surprise, virtually all the male participants seemed to enjoy experimenting with their feminine side (once they got over their initial resistance, of course). Clothes can provide a very physical anchor to how we feel. Wearing something that you have never worn before may have a big impact on your emotions and give you access to parts of you that you have rarely ever accessed. The key seems to be that if the woman is in charge of dressing the man, then it is not his fault he had to wear those sexy clothes *'and it actually doesn't feel that bad after all... Shhhh!'*

What was even more surprising to me is the large number of women that turned out to actually enjoy playing with full-size *Barbie* dolls. Raucous laughter ensues and, quite often, new sources of horniness can arise. It's all about how seriously do we take ourselves.

Women Wear Men's Clothes All the Time

Women seem to have become comfortable wearing men's clothes since about the Second World War, but for men, it is still highly controversial.[7] Compare a woman walking into a boardroom meeting in a nice and tight-

---

7. https://www.goodtherapy.org/blog/psychpedia/transvestite

ly tailored suit with a man walking into a boardroom meeting in a nice tight dress!

> *Without me having to initiate anything, she starts telling me what I should do and what I should wear. She even dresses me exactly to her liking, selecting each article of clothing and altering it if it's not exactly the way she wants it. She also knows what I like to see her wearing... and now she dresses me in a similar way. Simple, silky soft to the touch, with no distracting patterns or textures. Since she is telling me what to do, I can let go of any self-doubt and residual shame. I don't have to guess or figure things out for myself.*

> *She doesn't change her clothes. She doesn't need to. She is simply the dominant lesbian partner now... enjoying watching me and devouring me with her eyes. There is no doubt who is in charge.*

Lesbian Sex Anyone?

Most straight men (and women) love watching two hot girls kissing, making out and being sexual.[8] That's why some hetero-flexible women have fun making out with each other at a bar, knowing they are turning on the men they are trying to attract.[9]

While lesbian sex may be fun to watch, it can be far more fun (and edgy) to role-play. If virtual reality ever evolves to a full sensory experience to the point of being able to experience being inside someone else's body, how many people do you think would move from simply watching lesbian porn to enjoy experiencing being one of the girls? Sign me up! It might take a long time for that option to happen so, in the meantime, there is another option... It's super edgy and potentially shameful but really, isn't shame a party-pooper emotion that you would like to grow beyond?

> *Like most women, she has a potential bisexual side that we enjoy exploring. Perhaps, just the act of her being on top and taking the initiative is enough for some men to feel rejuvenated, but since I'm a little more uninhibited than most, I don't resist her inner lesbian desires to use clothing and lingerie to make me into her lesbian lover.*

> *'I want to see you more.' She puts one leg between mine and kicks my legs*

---

8. https://www.theatlantic.com/health/archive/2016/03/straight-men-and-lesbian-porn/472521/

9. https://www.psychologytoday.com/us/blog/power-and-prejudice/201207/girls-kissing-girls-0

apart before stepping back. 'Lean forward... lift your skirt a little more... walk over there... make me some tea while I watch you.'

Once she is finished observing me, the caressing starts, and she directs me to lie down.

The intimacy we experience in lesbian mode has a unique flavour that I never knew was possible before. Every touch, caress and (especially) the kissing is completely different...

After a while, I have had enough of receiving. Time to return the favour...

Photo credit: *StockSnap* (https://pixabay.com/users/stocksnap-894430/), https://pixabay.com/photos/jumper-cables-battery-engine-car-926308/

15

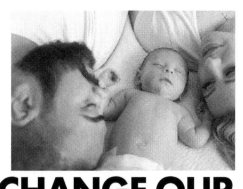

HAVING CHILDREN WILL NOT CHANGE OUR SEX LIFE

Harsh Reality of Parenting

Let's Hear It for the Mums

Let's start by acknowledging that none of us would be here without mothers and someone being in the nurturing role.[1] It's also likely to be the most tiring role most women will ever play in their lives. Let's hear it for the mums and their sacrifices!

Having said that, let's discuss the delicate matter of the mother role's shadow-side: Not being able to switch gears.[2] Just as some women get stuck in masculine mode and default to handling relationships in a controlled, business-like manner, the same can happen in mothering mode. It's understandable that when the survival of a dependant human relies on you that this can solidify your personality.[3,4]

1. https://www.nationalgeographic.com/news/2018/05/mothers-day-2018-maternal-instinct-oxytocin-babies-science/

2. https://www.hermeout.com/blog/mothering

3. https://www.theatlantic.com/health/archive/2015/01/what-happens-to-a-womans-brain-when-she-becomes-a-mother/384179/

4. https://www.thecut.com/2018/05/the-identity-transformation-of-becoming-a-mom.html

All Mum — All the Time

It's a widely-documented and well-known experience that when a woman becomes a mother, she often stops relating as wife/woman/lover in relation to her man.[5] For birth mothers, constant mothering is supported by hormones and aeons of survival conditioning. There is no blame or shame in this. It is totally normal.

Prior to having children, she may have been a horny, wild, carefree woman. After giving birth, her hormones switch her into nurturing mode. This is great because you want a mother to be naturally inclined to take care of her child and not out partying 'till the wee hours. In mother-mode, her hormones are going to make her feel non-sexual. As discussed earlier in this book, prolactin acts as a sexual breaker, and now she has prolactin on tap (so to speak) in the milk-production department. So guys, a word of advice: be patient and support her time of being non-sexual.

Where it does become a challenge is when the *'wife'* disappears for too long... perhaps more than 2 years after the birth of a child.

67% of couples had become very unhappy with each other during the first three years of their baby's life. Only 33% remained content. —Drs. John and Julie Gottman, Relationship Research Institute in Seattle.[6]

Viewing these statistics in light of the principles discussed in this book, we might have a framework to discuss new explanations, theories and solutions. For example, once a new baby arrives on the scene, a man often loses his only source of external feminine affection and the feel-good cuddling hormone—oxytocin. The mother, on the other hand, has an abundance of oxytocin from interacting with the child, breastfeeding and tactile support from girlfriends and mothers. For many people, physical affection may be a more important factor for a healthy relationship than sexual contact, so it's unrealistic to expect a relationship to survive forever in sensual isolation.

Men Also Love to Cuddle

Studies show that cuddling is an important factor in maintaining a solid relationship, and in general increases in importance in the later years of life.

---

5. https://www.psychologytoday.com/us/blog/the-second-noble-truth/201102/when-men-are-boys-and-wives-are-mothers

6. https://www.gottman.com/blog/bringing-baby-home-the-research/

Young couples worry if they aren't having enough sex, but physical intimacy plays an increasingly important role in keeping older couples together.[7]

A study by the Kinsey Institute involved 1,009 heterosexual *middle-aged* and *older* couples in long-term (average 25 years) committed relationships in five countries.[8] It showed an interesting reversal of stereotypes. *Kissing and hugging were more important to the happiness of [older] men than of women.*[9]

Thus it would seem that cuddling is not an optional extra that can be put off forever if you want the relationship to survive into old age.

One Modus Operandi

Anyway. Back to the present. Maybe you have a friend who is always in mother-mode. She seems to have an endless supply of wet wipes and granola bars in her cavernous handbag. She's a successful mother, so she tries to use her motherhood skills to achieve success in all realms. The problem is that you need different approaches to attack different life problems. If there are problems in the bedroom, the same motherhood suite of tools usually doesn't work so well on hubby.

So, it's great for women to be able to feel maternal, but when a woman spends 24/7 being in the *'spirit of all things maternal'* it can be difficult for her partner to penetrate her veil of motherhood in order to... well... putting it bluntly... penetrate her pussy. Especially if the control she needs to exert with her children transfers to her man and she starts to over-control or mother her husband.[10]

If you find that the constant mother-mode lasts for more than 2 years and you both are looking for a solution, there are things that you can do together to fix the situation. It's not impossible, but it does require commitment, practice, communication and a willingness to make it happen.

---

7. https://www.verywellmind.com/why-to-have-sex-more-often-2300937

8. Heiman, Julia R., et al. 'Sexual satisfaction and relationship happiness in midlife and older couples in five countries.' *Archives of sexual behavior* 40.4 (2011): 741-753.

9. http://healthland.time.com/2011/07/07/
    survey-shows-who-really-wants-to-cuddle-its-men/

10. https://www.verywellmind.com/parenting-your-spouse-is-not-okay-2302899

Schedule your Alone Time

It's a well-known trope in popular culture that when the magic in a long-term relationship disappears, couples fall into a rut and have sex routinely, once a week, whether they like it or not. But, is that such a bad idea? I mean, just because sex is part of your routine doesn't mean that the sex itself has to *be* routine. You can still have mind-blowing, deeply connected, heartfelt sex with multiple tantric orgasms if you schedule it for every *'Wicked Wednesday'* at 8pm.[11] Sometimes, even having fun takes discipline.[12]

People, especially parents, tend to act as though sex is a luxury item, like caviar or designer shoes, when in fact the Kinsey Report illustrated that most people described *'good sex'* as an essential component in creating a strong foundation for a satisfying relationship.[13]

Time for sex is often one of the first things to disappear when parents are trying to juggle their busy family life. It might not sound very sexy to schedule sex, especially as we got used to it happening organically by itself when the mood arose before the kids arrived. But let's face it, scheduled sex is probably better than unscheduled no-sex.

In a hectic household, who knows when the desire for sex and the capacity to have sex will occur simultaneously? Even if the moment arises, it may be all too short. A quickie in the bathroom after the kids go off to soccer practice may just not do it for you. Wouldn't it be way better to block out certain times of the week and dedicate that time to intimacy? Give yourselves some room in your schedule for sexy-time to happen.[14]

Even if the children are so young that you need to hire a babysitter, don't feel guilty about locking the door and telling the children *'This is Mummy and Daddy alone time. Only disturb us in a real emergency... such as if you have set yourself, the house or your sister on fire... OK?'*[15]

Children may well benefit from the healthy imprint of parents who have their own independent life together as man and woman. It may not be

11. https://www.huffpost.com/entry/marriage-and-sex-schedule-sex_n_1784519

12. https://www.health.com/sex/benefits-of-scheduling-sex

13. https://kinseyinstitute.org/pdf/ModernBride1949.pdf

14. https://www.psychologytoday.com/us/blog/fixing-families/201811/spontaneous-vs-scheduled-sex

15. https://www.huffingtonpost.com.au/sandra-pertot/why-your-sex-life-dies-when-kids-are-born_a_21577936/

a good imprint to constantly give the subliminal message that marriage equals no sex. I am not saying to have sex in front of them, only that you might be doing more harm than good if you hide the fact that sex is a natural thing. Kids are far more open-minded than we might give them credit for. Especially if affection has always been part of their normal, daily life.

Authentic Sexual Desire or the Biological Imperative?

Part of this parenting puzzle is to really, consciously plan *when* to have a child. Ideally, having another baby should be based on the feeling of love between the parents combined with other rational and logistical factors. Accidents and hormonal-driven outcomes are perhaps *not* the most conscious ways to make a baby, for the sake of everyone involved... especially the child.

The kind of sex that results from a mindless desire or an unspoken hope to keep a failing marriage together becomes a lot of unconscious pressure for a child. Wouldn't we all prefer to be born from loving and level-headed parents that really want us and at a time when they are as ready and prepared as they can be? But how do you know when you are really level-headed? There's an easy way to tell if your body is tricking your logical head into wanting more babies. If you suddenly become horny once a month, check out what time of your cycle that is. If thoughts of having another child occurs during the ovulation phase, your hormones might be driving that desire more than your rational mind.[16] If you become hornier during your menstrual cycle, it typically means that sub-consciously, you may not want a child as much as you thought.

One last point: If you have had a sexless marriage while your first child is growing and, all of a sudden, things become hot and horny, it might be your body yearning to breed again. Consider if now is the right time to have your next child or if you should use protection and enjoy your second honeymoon for a while longer.

Photo credit: *Stephanie Pratt* (https://pixabay.com/users/smpratt90-6113802/), https://pixabay.com/photos/family-newborn-baby-child-infant-2610205/

---

16. https://www.psychologytoday.com/us/blog/all-about-sex/201503/how-the-menstrual-cycle-affects-womens-libido

16
FAST IS BEST

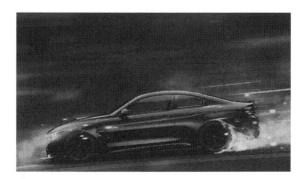

No Rabbits, Please

Ladies: how often have you found yourself in this scenario? You're with a male lover and the moment you give any indication that you might have just had an orgasm, he immediately starts pumping quickly, ejaculates and then rolls off of you? Being too fast is the most common complaint from women about men's sexual habits. The woman's preference is usually slower and with more variation. A study published in *The Canadian Journal of Human Sexuality* shows that when lesbians have sex, they spend roughly twice as much time in bed than heterosexual couples.[1,2,3]

In general, *'rabbit fuckers'* are the worst lovers. They only have one speed... high speed. The difficulty in addressing this means that many men *think* they are great in bed. Most of us probably found out the hard way that being honest with men about their sexual prowess can be a sex-killing move. Hence, the common practice of women faking orgasms.[4]

1. https://www.lehmiller.com/blog/2014/9/12/lesbians-may-have-sex-less-often-but-when-they-do-it-they-make-it-count

2. Blair, K.L. & Pukall, C.F. (2014). Can less be more? Comparing duration vs. frequency of sexual encounters in same-sex and mixed-sex relationships. *The Canadian Journal of Human Sexuality* 23:123–136; doi:10.3138/cjhs.2393 123

3. https://www.theguardian.com/lifeandstyle/2018/jul/09/do-lesbians-have-better-sex-than-straight-women

4. https://www.vice.com/en_us/article/pawmbg/married-women-orgasm-less-often-than-their-husbands-think-they-do

A Hard Man is Good to Find

Initiating sex with women is a lot of work. This is something I personally haven't done for a long time. First, you must chat them up, buy them drinks or dinner, convince them you're kind and a good talker. That already sounds like a lot of work but it gets much worse in the tantric situation. The man needs to invest at least one hour de-armouring her vagina, then her cervix (while she cries in pain), followed by sexually activating her spine, remove the shame of wanting to be slutty, talking her into a state beyond her normal contracted consciousness, teaching her to squirt, cervical orgasm and then finally do the equivalent of running a mini marathon to service the incredibly physically demanding womb orgasm. I get tired just typing it!

Before tantra, men chased women. After tantra, women seek out the few men capable of totally fulfilling the longing in a woman's body. Women actually seem more interested in sex than men if the quality is exceptional. Many things are backwards in the tantric world, including who chases whom. You can't believe the trouble I have got into from women that I wouldn't be in relationship with. Women don't seem to handle sexual rejection as well as men, who have been trained from an early age to deal with sexual rejection from women. If they can't have you some will even try and destroy you without even realising their subconscious motives. I learnt that the hard way from experience with seemingly sane past team members.

The New Tantra has trained several men to become professional tantric gigolos paid by women to perform tantric sex initiations (in countries where that isn't a problem). And, no, these clients aren't desperate women who have to resort to paying for it... quite the contrary. Most of them are beautiful, successful women at the top of their game who want to learn new skills and use their sexuality for more than just gratification. Often, the husband will pay big bucks for the session just to watch and learn. The best men like to learn and are humble enough to be coached.

It Takes Two Not to Tango

As we have discussed before, there is one major game-changer for men who want to raise their stock price in bed. Try to never ejaculate. You don't need to get religious about it, you will always have a few mistakes (misses) per year... just do your best to free yourself in relation to what is arguably the biggest addiction on this planet. I'm still working on it.

Practising tantra without the support of your partner is virtually impossible, so you might be wondering how to enlist your lover's support for your newfound tantric, non-ejaculating mission, especially when many women derive their self-esteem from making the man orgasm and see it as a lack of their skills and desirability if the man doesn't finish?[5,6] Even worse, feeling obligated to provide a sexual service without genuine interest and trying to get it over with as quickly as possible.

The answer to enlisting her help is to clearly communicate that you want to work at becoming a better lover, and that means learning how to slow down and not do the regular orgasm. If she asks why, just tell her it is because you adore her and want to have delicious sex with her for hours and to do so, you need to avoid cumming because, once you do, you will get sleepy and lose interest in sex. That level of honesty should do the trick! If not, it may take repetition and time for her to understand you are really committed to this practice. Once she gets to enjoy the fruits of your abstinence practice (namely, becoming a mindful lover who can have sex at a totally different level), you probably won't have to twist her arm for very long. If she doesn't want to support you and it's a high priority to improve yourself, you might be with the wrong woman.

Enlisting your partner's help also involves communicating with a new terminology in bed. *'Slowly!'* means *'Slow down right now, I am overheating!'* and *'Stop!'* means *'Don't breathe, don't wiggle and don't make a sound or it's all over!'* Make it unapologetically clear what the consequences will be of not working together as a team. It takes a lot of commitment to get out of the well-rehearsed routine of squeezing the bodily base to produce that pumping 5-second spasm orgasm, for both men and women.

Here's an example of how that conversation might go:

Your lover is in bed beside you, reading a book. Her hair is all messed up, and she's scrunching up her nose as she does when she's concentrating. She's wearing a sleeveless shirt that's a little too big for her and you get treated to a peek at her side-boob. What if you just rest your hand on her thigh, maybe massage her a bit, to see if she's willing to put down her novel? After a few minutes, she gets to a good place to take a break.

---

5. https://www.menshealth.com.au/women-love-watching-guys-ejaculate

6. https://www.betweenusclinic.com/premature-ejaculation/
    women-actually-drawn-men-premature-ejaculation/

FAST IS BEST

'Hey Honey, would you like to try something with me? I'd like to do a little tantric sex experiment from that weird new tantra book I've been reading. Would you like to give it a shot?'

'Oh, you mean trying all those weird Kama Sutra positions while we chant in the light of glowing candles and refer to our genitals as 'Yoni and Lingam'?'

'Ahhh... not exactly what I had in mind. It's not that kind of book... it's actually really practical and down to earth and one of the best sex books I've ever read, so you should rush out and buy a dozen copies for all your friends this Christmas. (Sorry! I couldn't resist putting a not-so-subliminal little advert in there). I just want to see what happens if we both build up our horniness and don't release it in our regular orgasm way. I heard interesting things can happen if you keep building up that energy indefinitely. Wanna try with me?'

'Sounds like we would miss the best part, but OK...' She looks perplexingly at you like you just told her that having diarrhoea in a wetsuit is invigorating.

As soon as the man decides to move away from goal-oriented sex, he will *have to* slow down, or he will still easily reach the point-of-no-return. In the beginning, he will undoubtedly have a *'miss'*. My advice: Don't beat yourself up if it really was an accident, but at the same time really check if there was a part of you that chose to cum. If you saw a subtle choice to go for the quick thrill, really spell out to yourself the cause and effect of that happening, and notice the short and any long-term negative effects that orgasm had on you. It is by understanding and realising the repercussions of the regular orgasm that will provide the fuel for change. Pain can be a great motivator. If it was just a simple lack of practice, don't sweat it. You've still taken another useful step towards developing new skills in bed that will accumulate over time. Think of it more akin to becoming a master golf player. It takes quite a lot of time to get really good at it, and there is never a point where self-mastery is complete. From my eyes, just that the man has the self-discipline and intention to become a better lover is in itself appealing.

Photo credit: *Parbol Studio* (https://www.shutterstock.com/g/ParabolStudio), https://www.shutterstock.com/image-illustration/high-speed-black-sports-car-street-727934728

17

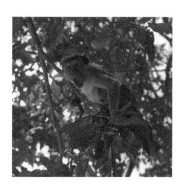

TO STOP EJACULATING, CLENCH

That Old 'Strangling the Monkey' Myth

Clenching the bodily base to stop ejaculating is the most common method recommended by Tantra and Tao teachers. The problem is that it won't allow the female consort to reach the deepest tantric orgasms. To really take her to the next level in the tantric elevator so to speak, you will need a more advanced technique. Tantric orgasms are just too horny for the man to *conduct* through his body when it is contracted. Let me explain using a car analogy for the guys. To get the clenching technique to work is like trying to push a car using the brake pedal. You have 2 opposing forces acting on each other. You can test it for yourself with a little experiment.

   Don't worry if you are reading this book at work. Drop your drawers right now and masturbate while clenching/contracting your bodily base. (That *was* a joke if your boss just walked in... anyway, back to our experiment.) Close your eyes and clench your bodily base right now as if you were masturbating or having sex. It doesn't matter if you are a man or a woman, it will have the same effect. If you are a human being, you will probably notice that stimulation increases as you clench, not decreases. In fact, it is a method to feel more sensation. So, if you are trying not to cum by clenching (and thereby making yourself hornier), you will be working against yourself. There is a better way, but it's more difficult to master.

The Relax and Conduct Method

If you want to master tantric sex to the level in which she can reach the highest tantric orgasm — the womb orgasm, you will need to learn how to be able to contain an extreme amount of horny sensations moving from her body into yours without going over the edge. In fact, you will need to be able to get to the (very rare) point of mastery where she trusts your capacity to keep going so that she can truly let go and (finally) stop withholding her sexual energy. She needs to feel free to fully explore and constantly generate huge amounts of sexual energy in an uninhibited way, without you losing it. Most women have been trained by thousands of less-than-perfect sexual encounters to perceive that really letting go equates to early termination of her most pleasurable moment. Finally, she is about to be guided beyond her masculine headspace of self-control and into her deepest free-fall... but if the guy can't handle those kilowatts of sexual energy she is producing, whah whah whaaaaah... Proceed to tantric jail and do not collect $200. This can be both frustrating for the woman and emasculating for the aspiring *'fully-in-control'* man.

With that dynamic in mind, it's no wonder lesser-men have traditionally tried to stifle women's full-blown sexuality. In tantra, the woman's body is seen as superior in sexual energy. TantraMan's job is to transcend the traditional temptation of instant gratification by expanding, merging with and conducting that force rather than limiting it, and then using it for spiritual growth/liberation. Something like the traditional explanation of the word *'tantra'*:

The word Tantra comes from the Sanskrit roots 'tanoti' meaning 'to expand' and 'trayati' meaning 'liberation'. The verbal root of tantra is √tan, 'to expand,' followed by the suffix ~tra, which is usually an instrumental suffix. Hence tantra means 'an instrument (tra) for expansion (tan)'[1]

Claro?

Same Goes for the Woman

The non-contracting technique is the same for the woman. When you are getting over-heated, relax. It is important for the woman to soften and relax because contracting a greedy pussy will make a man ejaculate real quick! Work as a team, my friends!

---

1. https://hareesh.org/blog/2015/6/10/definition-of-the-word-tantra

Ejaculation and orgasming on the pudendal nerve is usually initiated by contraction.[2] This is why in previous chapters, I recommended practising by masturbating with open legs and breathing regularly. A tantric woman can practise relaxing her vagina when she is really horny... kind of like reverse Kegels.[3]

Ping, Ping

Describing sensations in words is rarely easy. Here's another analogy to try to understand how the relaxation method works. Think of waves of pleasure as a kind of subtle sexual shockwaves. Imagine the woman's body producing a sort of sexual resonance wave that you feel as sexual electricity in your penis and bodily base. When that wave hits something hard and contracted in your body, it produces a very sharp and clear signal, and that signal is what sets off the pudendal nerve into a spasm orgasm. The contractions in the body (such as an anus tightened from tension and fear), not only reflects the signal back but also blocks the sexual stimulation from circulating freely. When sexual stimulation builds up and has nowhere else to go, the pudendal nerve goes into spasm. But if you don't have any contraction in your bodily base for the sexual stimulation signal to bounce off, no involuntary orgasm ensues. Problem solved! Simple... just not very easy!

It takes a lot of practice of self-witnessing your body to be able to detect the slightest contractions in your perineum area, while at the same time being present with your partner. Sex can become like an active meditation, a ruthless reality-checking meditation and one that you can't fake you have mastered.

Never Clench Then?

Does this mean you should never clench the bodily base? Not entirely. Contracting your bodily base initially can be a way to build up sexual stimulation faster. The next time you masturbate or have sex, pay close attention to what is happening down there. Chances are you habitually contract your bodily base to increase stimulation without realising it. There is nothing wrong with that at the start when you want to get horny and turn up the sexual heat. It's like kindling for a fire, but the trick is to pay close attention

---

2. https://onlinelibrary.wiley.com/doi/pdf/10.1111/j.1464-410X.2005.05536.x

3. https://www.healthline.com/health/fitness-exercise/reverse-kegel

to feel when the flame is getting too high and is about to combust your marshmallow into a crusty black blob of charcoal.[4]

When you want to be less turned on, you'll need to remember to switch from clenching to relaxing your taint.[5] If you don't, you may find yourself following the ingrained habit of contracting to spasm without even realising it. You've probably trained yourself to clench for however long you've been sexually active, so it will take some time to undo this habit. Being mindful is the first step in breaking any habit. Instead of checking out in a fantasy, just focus on the pure physical sensations. The longer time since your last 'miss', the more sexual energy you will have (and be able) to conduct around your body.[6]

I will cover the technique to move energy around your body in the next chapter. The more you progress at 'circulating energy',[7] the more your tantric lover will grow in confidence and your ability to conduct her horniness and allow her the opportunity to surrender and unleash her most intense sexual energy. It's quite a spectacle to watch... let alone to be plugged into! Game on?

Photo credit: *PublicDomainPictures* (https://pixabay.com/users/publicdomainpictures-14/), https://pixabay.com/photos/monkey-screaming-yelling-loud-wild-20182/

---

4. https://www.healthline.com/health/healthy-sex/is-edging-bad#potential-benefits

5. https://www.nafc.org/bhealth-blog/how-to-relax-your-pelvic-floor

6. https://www.healthline.com/health/healthy-sex/semen-retention#research

7. The g-tummo meditative practice targeted at controlling 'inner energy' is described by Tibetan practitioners as one of the most sacred spiritual practices in the Indo-Tibetan traditions of Vajrayana Buddhism and Bon. It is also called 'psychic heat' practice since it is associated with descriptions of intense sensations of bodily heat in the spine. Kozhevnikov M, Elliott J, Shephard J, Gramann K (2013) *Neurocognitive and Somatic Components of Temperature Increases during g-Tummo Meditation: Legend and Reality.* PLoS ONE 8(3): e58244. https://doi.org/10.1371/journal.pone.0058244

18

PREMATURE EJACULATION IS UNCONTROLLABLE

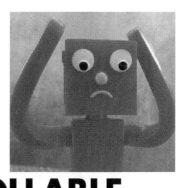

Not So Fast!

Even if you suffer from the kind of premature ejaculation that Hollywood teen jock movies make fun of, there are tantric techniques that really work, even where traditional methods fail.[1] So, fear not if you're an unwilling member of the Rapid-Uncontrollable-Genital-Sneeze club. Your situation is only temporary, and help is on its way! In fact, you can regain full control in a matter of days. A big claim, I know! But over the course of 10 years, I have seen it happen to countless workshop participants. This might sound too good to be true, and in the sexology world, it would be... but that is because traditional sexual practices don't understand techniques for circulating sexual energy.

How to Circulate Sexual Stimulation

De-armour your Anus

In Chapter 10, I explained how and why it might be good sexual practice to de-armour your ass. If you need to revisit this concept or if you also have the memory of a goldfish (like yours truly... what was I saying?), now is the time to grab some lube and give it a try. You'll need to have a de-armoured ass if you are going to move sexual energy backwards and

---

1. IMDB:Most Popular Premature Ejaculation, Teenage Boy Feature Films, https://www.imdb.com/search/keyword/?keywords=premature-ejaculation%2Cteenage-boy&sort=moviemeter,asc&mode=detail&page=1&title_type=movie&ref_=kw_ref_typ

away from the penis towards your spine.

De-armouring is complete when the man can feel pleasure in his ass. This is because there needs to be a *'bridge'* of pleasurable flesh between your penis and your tailbone. Think of this as sexual yoga. If one part of that bridge is tightly contracted in residual fear, it will act as a roadblock.[2] If your ass is contracted, the sexual stimulation will just get trapped at the front of the body. Something I suspect is not the best option for long-term men's health.

Once the anus is able to feel sexual pleasure, sexual stimulation will move back towards the spine *by itself*. No visualising or other techniques are needed. This is the difference between this technique and others.

If you still have *'ass shame'*, try to convince yourself while you are *'putting from the rough'* that you are doing it purely for altruistic motives. You're learning how to be a better lover for your partner's sake right? My point is, don't feel guilty.[3] Practice makes perfect. Eventually, sandpaper friction and discomfort will morph into slippery backdoor pleasure, and you may find that the uncontrollable reflex of the spasm orgasm miraculously recedes into the background.

Sexually Activate Your Spine

If your spine is sexually activated, sexual stimulation will hit the base of the spine and naturally and effortlessly move upwards, making the torso undulate. It can feel like a series of waves that move along your spine. Unlike the de-armouring process, which is easy to explain and replicable at home, it's impossible to sexually activate your spine through reading a book. (Sorry, no refunds!) All I can tell you is that in The New Tantra level 1 sexual de-conditioning workshop,[4] through a process of breathing exercises and becoming vulnerable, the spine can be sexually activated in about 80% of people. The result is that it looks like the person's spine moves like an undulating snake. Perhaps that's one of the meanings of the whole kundalini snake story. It's a one-off-process, so

---

2. https://www.huffpost.com/entry/hidden-tensions-that-take_b_5741432

3. Branfman, Jonathan, Susan Stiritz, and Eric Anderson. 'Relaxing the straight male anus: Decreasing homohysteria around anal eroticism.' *Sexualities* 21.1-2 (2018): 109-127.

4. https://www.thenewtantra.com/

once it is done, you won't need to be initiated again. I know it sounds kind of woo-woo-weirdo-positive-thinking-huffy-fluffy-tantric-bullshit when you haven't experienced it for yourself, but it's actually quite down-to-earth and not that strange when you feel it in your own body.

The Most Dangerous Minutes

Be extra careful at the start because those first few minutes of sexual activity are the most dangerous.[5] The ability to conduct the sexual energy around the body increases minute by minute and also day after day since your last 'miss'. Therefore, take a few short breaks at the start.[6,7]

Even 30 seconds of no movement is often enough to calm things down. Keep things cool and monitor your horniness in percentages, and stay below 80% to the point of no return. This means avoiding the temptation to feel the really warm, buzzing, horny sensations by getting too horny and pushing yourself beyond your limit... or trying to please your partner and proving you are a good lover. Remember: crying out 'Stop!' signals when you are rapidly approaching the edge, but it can also be seen as a war-cry, signifying that you are seriously committed to fighting the spasm orgasm reflex.

Photo credit: *Erika Wittlieb* (https://pixabay.com/users/erikawittlieb-427626/), https://pixabay.com/photos/upset-sad-confused-figurine-534103/

5. https://www.nhs.uk/conditions/ejaculation-problems/

6. https://lifehacker.com/how-men-can-last-longer-during-sex-1829473619

7. Martin, Christopher, et al. 'Current and emerging therapies in premature ejaculation: Where we are coming from, where we are going.' *International Journal of Urology* 24.1 (2017): 40-50.

19

ERECTILE DYSFUNCTION COMES WITH AGE

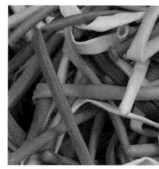

Natural Viagra

Is a soft cock just something that we should expect and accept with old age?[1] Should we plan a retirement of shopping with our old folks' cards for hearing aids, batteries, adult diapers and Viagra? After all, there are studies like the *Massachusetts Male Ageing Study* that demonstrate that erectile dysfunction (ED) is increasingly prevalent with age. At age 40, approximately 40% of men are affected. The rate increases to nearly 70% of men aged 70 years.[2] But correlation does not prove causation. Let's take a silly example to illustrate this point. Let's say 99% of cheerleaders that have back injuries were also reported to have used pompoms in their life, this doesn't mean that pompoms cause back injuries.

Although many risk factors for ED have been identified, such as age and obesity (which coincidentally are also risk factors for back injuries among cheerleaders), there may be other causes that have not yet been identified.[3] Certainly age is a factor in ED in a normal sexual lifestyle, but perhaps changing sexual practices may lessen the impact of age.

1. https://www.healthline.com/health/erectile-dysfunction/is-it-inevitable

2. Impotence and its medical and psychosocial correlates: results of the Massachusetts Male Aging Study. J. Urol., 151 (1994) https://www.ncbi.nlm.nih.gov/pubmed/8254833

3. https://www.mayoclinic.org/diseases-conditions/erectile-dysfunction/symptoms-causes/syc-20355776

All out of Ojas?

In traditional Tantra and Taoism, there are teachings that humans are born with a finite amount of sexual energy called *ojas*.[4] They say that energy is depleted through the regular orgasm. Those teachings aren't really very useful, as they cannot be proven scientifically, but what I kept hearing is that men reported they were being cured of ED by adopting tantric practices. It's probably due to the fact that we become more sensitive and more full of sexual energy the longer we don't orgasm *if* we keep sexually active.

If you've been reading this book from the beginning (and thus have proven you have the mental resilience to withstand silly Australian humour), then what I'm about to share with you will be of no surprise. These practices can virtually eliminate ED and give you back the ability to hoist ye ol' *'good wood'* on demand.

Most men realise it's harder to get horny or maintain an erection if you have recently had an ejaculation. I already mentioned the testosterone rebound after 7 days post-orgasm and the rat studies that suggest it can take as long as 15 days for the effects of orgasm exhaustion to disappear completely.[5,6]

Stop Trying to Be Someone Else

If you wake up with erections, can easily get them through masturbation, but have erectile difficulty with your partner, this points more towards psychological issues such as sexual shame or lack of attraction.[7] The litmus test is to check next time you are doing it solo and see if there is a difference between what you masturbate to and what you encounter in your regular sexual diet. Let me explain this in a little more detail.

If you are queer or kinky and you haven't fully come to terms with who you are and what makes you hot, then you probably already have your answer but maybe aren't willing to accept it. Most of us were taught by

---

4. Jordens, J. (1998). *Gandhi's Religion: A Homespun Shawl* (p. 26)

5. Jackson, S.B., Dewsbury, D.A. Recovery from sexual satiety in male rats. *Animal Learning & Behavior* 7, 119–124 (1979) https://doi.org/10.3758/BF03209668

6. https://www.menshealth.com/sex-women/a19524569/refractory-period/

7. Feldman HA, Goldstein I, Hatzichristou DG, et al: Impotence and its medical and psychosocial correlates: Results of the Massachusetts Male Aging Study. *J Urology*, 1994;151:54–61.

less-than-sexually-enlightened role models to be ashamed of our sexuality.[8] This is a good time to remember the saying by Dr Seuss, *Those who mind don't matter... and those who matter don't mind.* If you have a partner that truly loves you, maybe they are more willing to fully embrace your naughty sides than you imagine. If not, Dr Seuss-ify your life, maybe?

You are the designer of your sex life, so get in touch with what turns you on and support the Southern Regions (so long as it is between consenting adults that is). If you are totally bored with vanilla sex, leave the missionary position for... well, the missionaries? It may seem like common sense, but if you can stop judging yourself and talk honestly with your lover about what you like in bed, then you may find that your hard-ons and sexual appetite reappear.

But what if you have genuinely lost attraction to your partner? This is a big topic that we will cover in more detail over the next few chapters.

Photo credit: *Alicja* (https://pixabay.com/users/_alicja_-5975425/),
https://pixabay.com/photos/balloons-colorful-the-background-4243065/

---

8. Downs, A. (2005). *The Velvet Rage: Overcoming the Pain of Growing Up Gay in a Straight Man's World.* Da Capo Press.

20
MONOGAMY IS DIFFICULT

There May Be a Hidden Dividing Mechanism

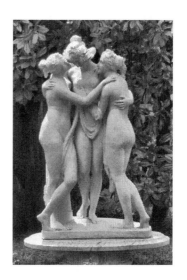

Remember that weeklong vacation you planned with your lover that you anticipated for months? The first two days were great. You had sex all over the cabin. Not a piece of furniture was safe from your sexual antics. But how long can you keep going like that? You might notice the short-term effect of orgasming quite easily, but in the long-term, how long does the honeymoon hyper-sex frequency continue?[1] Review your past experience from your own life with this perspective in mind and you might see a more universal pattern that we all experience.

Statistically it seems that holding a relationship together has never been more difficult.

In that study which involved 19,065 people during a 15-year period, rates of infidelity among men were found to have risen from 20 to 28%, and rates for women, 5 to 15%. ... Studies suggest around 30–40% of unmarried relationships and 18–20% of marriages see at least one incident of sexual infidelity.[2]

According to the famous relationship therapist Esther Perel one of the principal causes of the rate of infidelity rising is because of the ever

---

1. https://www.psychologytoday.com/us/blog/the-intelligent-divorce/201806/is-too-much-sex-possible

2. https://en.wikipedia.org/wiki/Infidelity

increasing demands that we put on one person to fulfil so many desires.[3]

And then we added romantic needs to the pairing, the need for belonging and for companionship. We have gone up the Maslow ladder of needs, and now we are bringing our need for self-actualisation to the marriage. We keep wanting more. We are asking from one person what once an entire village used to provide.[4]

I will leave the relationship coaching to the experts and concentrate on the sexual/biological components that are at play in this hot topic.

Orgasm Biology

Guys, remember how you feel in relation to your partner after you ejaculate, and answer this question honestly (I have asked thousands of men this question, and they all give the same response... when no woman is within earshot that is). *'Does she become more or less attractive to you after you cum?'* Sorry, ladies... The answer is a pretty universal *'less!'*[5] It seems that ejaculation has a built-in, biologically-programmed response to spread our oats around by making our partners less attractive once we orgasm.

Let's take a look at nature again to see if there are any clues as to whether our biological impulses support monogamy. You've probably heard it before, but there are many bonding-pair birds that mate for life. According to the *Sibley Guide to Bird Life and Behaviour*, 90% of all bird species are *socially but not sexually* monogamous.[6] This is an interesting distinction, as it means that although they stay together for many years (or even for life), they still occasionally breed with other birds to widen their gene pool. When botanists study avian DNA or observe their annual mating rituals, they find that socially monogamous birds will occasionally mate with other birds outside of their bonding pair. It is not uncommon for a male to be unknowingly rearing eggs in his nest that do not belong to him. Open-relationships of the feathered kind! But why would nature do this?

The reason is that if a species of birds was strictly monogamous, it would be evolutionarily less successful than those that aren't, because if

---

3. https://www.youtube.com/watch?v=P2AUat93a8Q

4. https://www.newyorker.com/culture/the-new-yorker-interview/
    love-is-not-a-permanent-state-of-enthusiasm-an-interview-with-esther-perel

5. https://www.irishtimes.com/life-and-style/health-family/
    my-boyfriend-loses-interest-in-sex-after-he-orgasms-1.3501903

6. https://www.birdwatchersdigest.com/bwdsite/solve/faqs/do-birds-mate-for-life.php

one partner was sterile, that would mean the end of two birds' breeding capacity. From a purely biological perspective, lifelong monogamy is a less than optimal strategy. Putting all your eggs in one basket (so to speak), is not the wisest strategy if you want to maximise the chances of your genetic material being passed along.

What's the Implication?

So, what does this practically mean to us? Is nature giving us the justification to be unfaithful? Should we all run around, sowing our seeds willy-nilly because nature has programmed us this way? This might sound like a fun excuse but maybe this program needs a 2.0 update. Don't you think there are enough humans on the planet from an environmental perspective?

Monogamy is arguably the deepest, cleanest, least dramatical and most practical way to go deep. It also wastes the least amount of resources to remain with one partner instead of constantly fighting the competition. So why then does it seem so difficult for many people to stay monogamous?

Orgasming repeatedly through the pudendal nerve may be unconsciously putting us into *'bring me a fresh one'* mode. The scientific term for this phenomenon in animals is the *'Coolidge effect'*. It's described as a situation in which a partner, usually a male, wants to have sex with a new mate and they lose interest in their prior sexual partner.[7,8,9,10] We are talking about animals here, right?

The President and Mrs. Coolidge were being shown around an experimental government farm. When she came to the chicken yard she noticed that a rooster was mating very frequently. She asked the attendant how often that happened and was told, 'Dozens of times each day.' Mrs. Coolidge said, 'Tell that to the President when he comes by.' Upon being told, Coolidge asked, 'Same hen every time?' The reply was, 'Oh no, Mr. President, a different hen every time.' Coolidge: 'Tell that to Mrs. Coolidge!' —Professor of Psychology Frank

7. https://en.wikipedia.org/wiki/Coolidge_effect

8. Brown, R. E. (1974), 'Sexual arousal, the Coolidge effect and dominance in the rat (Rattus norvegicus)', *Animal Behaviour*, 22 (3): 634–637, doi:10.1016/S0003-3472(74)80009-6

9. Lester, GL; Gorzalka, BB (1988), 'Effect of novel and familiar mating partners on the duration of sexual receptivity in the female hamster', *Behavioral Neural Biology*, 49 (3): 398–405, doi:10.1016/s0163-1047(88)90418-9, PMID 3408449

10. Pinel, J. (2007), *Biopsychology* (6th ed.) ISBN 0-205-42651-4

A. Beach, responsible for the introduction of the term *'Coolidge Effect'*.[11]

Without self control, our ancient brain, the reptilian brain, can override our logical pre-frontal cortex and urge us to compulsively spread our genes around. Indulging in the spasm orgasm may exacerbate this internal tug-of-war between our instinctive impulses and how we would like to behave. In other words, our higher self may want intimacy and commitment, but our instincts are prodding us to find someone new to have sex with, moved by the mistaken biological memory that we are still fighting sabre-tooth tigers at lunch, and bubonic plague on the weekend.

Temporary Honeymoon

So, coming back to our cabin sex example. How often were you having sex in your honeymoon periods? 2-4 times a day? And, how long was it before that frequency started to diminish? About three months or so? If you are like most of us, you have probably experienced a similar story. This may explain why girls were traditionally told by worried mothers to not let the man *'have his way'* before marriage.[12] The short-term effects are fairly obvious to most women who are experienced in the dating game with men.

So, the answer seems fairly simple, if you analyse it: Don't trigger this biological repelling mechanism. People who practise sexual continence of not orgasming on the pudendal nerve (both men and women), usually find that the attraction does not diminish in the same way as it does with the normal sexual lifestyle. Indulging in the pudendal orgasm might have a higher cost than you bargained for. Furthermore, people who stay sexually active while refraining from the pudendal nerve orgasm often report they *regain* lost sexual attraction to their long-term partner.

It seems that not activating primal separation signals in the first place may be a better strategy to outsmart that silly old reptilian brain than trying to use mental rationale to override it after the fact.

Photo credit: *JamesDeMers* (https://pixabay.com/users/jamesdemers-3416/), https://pixabay.com/photos/statue-marble-sculpture-53783/

---

11. https://medium.com/moments-of-passion/
    why-sex-becomes-mind-numbingly-boring-daad10dcb7

12. https://goodmenproject.com/featured-content/why-buy-the-cow-hgraylicsw/

21

INFIDELITY RUINS RELATIONSHIPS

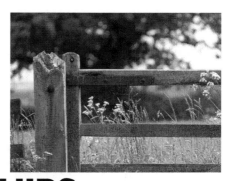

Greener Grass

Probably, most people in society would agree with this one. Without a doubt, very few of us have escaped the pain of sexual or emotional betrayal. Maybe it brings back a painful memory of a *'sext'* that you saw over your supposedly monogamous partner's shoulder, or a phone call you overheard. Sometimes, you just sense the unspoken reason why your lover has become distant or why they started acting weird, for no apparent reason. The most extreme scenario is that you actually catch them in bed together with someone else.

In this scenario, a violent, uncontrollable reaction is so socially acceptable that in the U.S., France, Australia and several other countries, there is often a *'heat of passion'* defence that can be raised in a court of law in murder cases.[1,2,3] If someone comes home to find their lover in bed with another person, grabs the kitchen knife and filets them, they could raise this as a legitimate defence in court.[4] What might have been a murder verdict can be reduced to manslaughter.[5] So, the concept that a relationship will be ruined by the betrayal of having an affair, and that our reaction to it will

---

1. https://www.merriam-webster.com/legal/heat%20of%20passion
2. https://www.telegraph.co.uk/news/uknews/law-and-order/9020632/Crimes-of-passion-defence-restored-in-murder-cases.html
3. http://www5.austlii.edu.au/au/legis/qld/consol_act/cc189994/s304.html
4. https://www.lacriminaldefenseattorney.com/legal-dictionary/c/crime-of-passion/
5. https://www.justia.com/criminal/docs/calcrim/500/570/

be uncontrollable, is deeply embedded in most societies across the globe.

Sometimes You're the Baby, Sometimes You're the Diaper

Some of us have experienced this as both victim and perpetrator. Others have only experienced one side or the other, but it's a lose-lose situation for both sides. Even if you're the cheater, you're hopefully struggling with your conscience. The tug-of-war between desiring a new lover and the fear of losing the relationship you already have, is probably fairly familiar to many of us. Perhaps you don't want to deal with the pain that comes with telling your lover the truth. You might build a web of deceit and erect an invisible barrier between your partner and yourself, and destroy intimacy as a result.

If you discover you are the one being cheated upon, your ego may be crushed, and you feel hurt because your partner doesn't find you attractive any more. The insecurity, fear and anger that goes with being cheated on is an endless source of material for both Bollywood and Hollywood because it can cut to our very core of our belief in others and even ourselves. It hurts to learn that you can't trust your partner and even more to feel the disrespect of having been lied to and taken for a fool.[6] You may feel like the relationship is unsalvageable because you can't trust your partner anymore, so you end it... and, if you don't, your friends see you as a doormat.

This being the case, why would anyone risk trying anything else? The answer is because many people long for non-monogamy... and that ideal of having an open-relationship is growing. Yougov conducted a survey that was mentioned in the Monogamy episode of the Netflix series, *Explained*.[7,8] In this survey of one thousand Americans, roughly 30% of adults revealed that their ideal relationship would involve some degree of non-monogamy. What wasn't mentioned is that in that same survey, when you look at the segment of people under 30 years of age, the percentage of people who long for some degree of non-monogamous relationship jumps to about

---

6. https://www.psychologytoday.com/us/blog/the-mysteries-love/201601/why-is-infidelity-so-painful

7. YouGov, Relationships Survey, (September 23–25, 2016). Question 1. Ideal Relationship, https://d25d2506sfb94s.cloudfront.net/cumulus_uploads/document/cqmk3va41c/tabs_OP_Relationships_20160925.pdf

8. Netflix, Explained, Season 1, Episode 3, Monogamy https://www.imdb.com/title/tt8449054/?ref_=ttep_ep3

50%. So, one out of two people under 30 years old is willing to admit that they desire some kind of open relationship... at least in theory.

Let's be totally clear on this point, I am not advocating infidelity, nor do I believe that an open-relationship is somehow superior to monogamy. In fact, an open relationship is probably not the most appropriate option for most couples. We're just discussing different options here. Ok?

Different Strokes

Obviously, there is no one-rule-for-all-the-people. Someone who switches partners too easily may grow more by staying with one person through difficult times. Fear of commitment and intimacy may drive an impulse to nit-pick and find faults in partners, and then use those faults as justification to leave the relationship too easily. You probably have met someone like this. Every time you see them, they have a new lover on their arm. Sometimes they date someone who is clearly a hot mess, but even when they are dating someone who suits them really well, you know it's not worth it to get attached or accept their social media friend request because they are not going to be around for very long. In the end, that friend might say something like, 'You know I can't be tied down.' They feel trapped by the commitment and scoff at the work involved in creating intimate relationships. However, monogamy may be just what the doctor ordered for this kind of person to grow. Different people and different situations require different solutions.

Love Vs Fear

Monogamy is clearly the best option in many circumstances. When two people fall in love, there is a natural loss of interest in others. Love-based sex is undoubtedly deeper than sex without feelings and couples deeply in love generally don't have the same need for self-control as there is a natural loss of interest in chasing others when one is satisfied and consumed with their partner. This is what I term *love-based monogamy*.

What I see many unhappy couples get stuck in, is a different thing altogether: *fear-based monogamy*. This is when one partner loses interest in having sex with the other, and then employs guilt and fear to trap the other into sexual abstinence. Yes, it's the usually accepted way, but it might not be the highest/most unconditionally loving option. The emotional safety of conventional fear-based monogamy may well be easier than the alternative, but it often comes at the cost of a sexless relationship.

We'll cover the whole jealousy issue in a lot more detail in the next chapter.

Longings and Fantasies

I have a working theory that sexual fantasies are indicators of the strongest way to awaken life-energy in the body. For this reason, suppressing our sexual sub-conscious may also sap our vital energy and lock us into living in an unauthentic way. Pretending we don't have our dirty little fantasies is the status quo in our sex-shaming society. Perhaps, there is a bigger cost than just creating a fake persona; we might also be blocking ourselves from deeper personal development and potential in the form of freeing up mental attention.

The Freedom *From* Longing

Imagine feeling a relaxed, horny energy in your body but without the incessant, distracting fantasies popping into your head. I call that state *mental celibacy*.

The way to become mentally celibate permanently is to act out all your fantasies in a tantric way. Eventually, when you have physically experienced your fantasies at maximum horniness for long enough, you naturally stop thinking about those acts when they're not happening. When mental celibacy is achieved, it is such a relief to be able to use that energy to focus on more productive tasks. You might still consciously *choose* to think about those fantasies, but the *compulsion* has gone.

The problem is that very few people seem to get horny or masturbate to monogamy *unless* they have lived out their group-sex fantasies. Sex with multiple partners at the same time, or sex with people other than your partner are the most common fantasies, but once you have lived out those fantasies fully, the allure seems to disappear and generally loses its power to distract you from what you actually have. In a nutshell, it's far easier to be satisfied with one person once you are out the other end of the fantasy tunnel. Sex with the same person becomes more satisfying as FOMO (fear of missing out) subsides, and the forbidden fruit loses its allure once truly enjoyed. The problem is, for most of us, there's no simple shortcut through mental acrobatics by trying to jump over the *doing* part.

Wake Up or Fake Out

A good way to shut down sexual energy is to pretend that you don't want what you want. Good girls don't want gang bangs; so many women with this fantasy experience shame and hide this very common female fantasy, not knowing how normal that actually is. Having heard thousands of fantasies during the hundreds of workshops I conducted, this is one of the most common. The other one I rarely hear sexually liberated women *not* having is the girl-on-girl fantasy. Domination and submission are right up there too. So, if we're in a strictly monogamous relationship, how could we possibly fulfil those fantasies? The threesome fantasy, sex with a stranger, group sex and bisexual fantasies are all logistically impossible.

Infidelity does not break marriages up; it is the unreasonable expectation that a marriage must restrict sex that breaks a marriage up. One of the reasons I wrote the book is that I've seen so many long-term relationships broken up simply because one had sex outside the relationship. But feeling victimised isn't a natural outcome of casual sex outside a relationship; it is a socialised victimhood. I'm not advocating cheating; I'm advocating open and equitable sexual relationships. —Eric Anderson, American sociologist and sexologist

If you both do decide you want to venture into these hazardous waters, how could you open up your relationship? Very carefully, is my advice!

Open Relationship Pointers

Here are some suggested guidelines that may be helpful. These are not rules, but pointers that many people have found useful but, caveat utilitor, you will have to tailor this advice to suit your situation, openness and you and your partner's limits:

1. **Communicate:** Start by asking if your partner wants to hear your fantasies. I am surprised to see how many people tell me that they don't know what their partner masturbates to. This can be a very liberating exercise in itself. For example, try walking down the street and discretely play the game of pointing out people you find attractive and what you would like to do with them. You may be surprised to find that you share the same taste and creative ideas. Even if nothing ever materialises from it, it can be quite a horny game and also helps *'keepin' it real'* between each other. It's only natural to be attracted to others. Bravery and honesty may lead to a much deeper level of trust

between you (but it may also put the nails in the coffin of an already doomed relationship). Imagine the relaxation that may accompany you saying, *'Yes, I am attracted to that person, but I am choosing you as my long-term partner.'* That's a compliment you can bank on! We all know there will always be someone younger, hotter, more charismatic or with a bigger *'member'*. Pretending that this is not true only makes our bullshit detectors beep loudly and distrust our partner's fake assurances to the contrary. Realise there is a *big* difference between someone you would have a *'roll in the hay'* with and someone you want to invest time and effort in to grow with as a life partner.

2. **Set an Intention:** Do you intend to make your primary relationship stronger by introducing someone else, or are you using a 3rd person to escape from the real issues at hand? Don't open your relationship when things are bad between your partner and yourself. Remember, the grass always *appears* to be greener over that damn fence. New relationship energy can only be a crutch for so long. Eventually, you'll be able to see that the same shortcoming that led your current relationship to stall, may cause your new relationship to fail as well. The novelty of *newness* is always alluring, and the idea of being found attractive is certainly highly intoxicating. Be honest with yourself and your partner regarding your motivation to experiment.[9] Do you truly want to enhance your current relationship? If so, the shared novelty of experimental play with others can certainly inject fresh energy into a diminished sex life. Many couples think they'd quite like to have a beautiful, (and possibly younger) partner (usually a woman) who is single and wants to be part of their sexual landscape. The object of this fantasy is called a *'sexual unicorn'* because they are so rare. Relatively few young bisexual women want to play sexually with an older and already established couple who have lost sexual interest in each other and need her around as a catalyst to rekindle their fire. Of those who are sexually interested in this kind of relationship, even fewer have the skills to develop and maintain such a relationship.

3. **Transparency:** Before you do anything, ask your partner for permission about every detail of the grey areas. Don't use vagueness to your ad-

---

9. https://www.psychologytoday.com/us/blog/love-without-limits/201008/why-do-people-choose-polyamory

vantage. Be honest and transparent, and tell the other everything they would like to know. This includes talking to your partner about your feelings. Keep the interaction with the 3rd person clean and within the parameters of the agreement. For instance, do not secretly send texts or emails if you have agreed not to. Keep asking yourself whether you would like your partner to do what you are considering doing. You will probably need to think and talk through all of the concerns about opening up the relationship. Transparency and honesty make things simpler... at least in your head.

4. **Invite someone else into your bed, together:** Don't go off by yourself... at least until there is well-established trust between you. Bringing another woman into bed is the classic fantasy, but usually, it only works well if the man can fully satisfy one woman first. Inviting a man into a heterosexual couple's bed is usually much simpler. The men get to share the workload, experience non-competitive brotherhood and a chance to work through any possible homophobia issues. It's not required that the men touch each other (although that may be her wish)!

5. **Sexually-transmitted diseases:** Be highly responsible regarding the STD status of the individuals involved. If you and your partner have *really* been monogamous for a long time and were tested before you became fluid-bonded, only then you can be certain of your STD status. If you plan to introduce a new person into the mix, it's nice for everyone to get re-tested and show your results to the others. If a new person has not been tested for all STDs, you should still get tested again (even if you use condoms), roughly every three to six months after having sex with someone new because there is no such thing as 100% safe sex; only *safer* sex. Being sloppy with STD's is often one of the biggest legitimate reasons to end the open relationship experiment.

6. **Therapy:** Make sure you have some good therapy tools to deal with any of the insecurities that will probably come up. Do you know how to release your anger so that it doesn't turn into passive aggression? Do you have the skills to be able to confess the insecurities that arise inside of you? Most likely, you will need all the tools in your self-development box to benefit from turning this delicate stone over.

7. **Open Dating:** Eventually, if you are both in a good space together and you have both proven your trustworthiness to each other, *then* you might be ready to fly solo on an external date. This requires a high degree of confidence, self-worth and security in the knowledge that you have something solid with your partner. Afterwards, share your experience in as much detail as your partner wishes to hear.

8. **Respect:** Good manners and respect can go a long way in such delicate situations. If you were to borrow a car from a friend and you would fill up the tank, wash it and say *'thank you'* when you return it, you would probably have a much higher chance of a repeated lending offer plus a stronger relationship with the lender. While a relationship is not the same as the one-way ownership of a car, there are some similarities. A call of *'thanks for lending me your partner last night, I really appreciate it. Is there anything you would like to talk over?'* can be one of the strongest ways to display the lack of intention to *compete* between people, and show respect at the same time. Three people working towards the same goals can be a truly liberating experience.

Let's continue this topic and discuss in further detail the main reason for not opening up a relationship... jealousy.

Photo credit: *Kevin* (https://pixabay.com/users/kevsphotos-3037209/), https://pixabay.com/photos/farm-gate-countryside-landscape-1591383/

22

JEALOUSY = LOVE

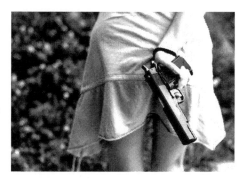

Practising Unconditional Love

Jealousy and monogamy are the most charged areas of sexuality and hence I am devoting 2 chapters to these overlapping topics. Let's go into more detail and explore the dynamics of jealousy.

In long-term monogamous relationships, it is common to find the paradigm of: *'I love you, so I don't want to share you. Even if I am not interested in having sex with you anymore, you sure as hell can't have sex with anyone else... because I love you!'*

Although this is pretty much the norm, isn't it illogical if we really analyse it deeply? If one person is not interested in an activity, why would they deny the other the opportunity and thus have them suffer?[1] Easy if the issue is bowling, but as soon as we involve sex, things become clouded by emotions. Isn't withholding more akin to acting with self-interest because we do not have the *capacity* to love unconditionally?[2] If we truly, unconditionally loved our partner but did not want to have sex with them, what would be the logical thing to do? Wouldn't we want to see them happy if we had the altruism of a saint and could handle the strong emotions of jealousy? If we could really operate from our most loving self, wouldn't we perhaps arrange for a trusted person to serve their needs if it was done in a respectful manner?

Cases of terminal illness, combined with the loss of sexual ability, seems

1. https://www.psychologytoday.com/us/blog/close-encounters/201410/
whats-really-behind-jealousy-and-what-do-about-it

2. https://www.mindbodygreen.com/0-4171/Unconditional-Love-How-to-Give-It-and-How-to-Know-When-Its-Real.html

to grant some a higher perspective.[3] They set their partner up with a new person to be their companion, lover and support before and after the traumatic experience of death. But what if we were able to do this under less extreme circumstances?

Friends Vs Lovers

Why is it that we often treat our partners worse than we do our close friends? Let me elaborate. Do we try to control our friends' sex lives? (If you do, you are probably reading the wrong book :p) Why then don't we give the same courtesy to someone just because we have rubbed genitals with them? Why should the first person arriving at the scene have rights over the second? There must be other reasons behind restraining our sexual desires so strongly.

Mimetic Desire

According to René Girard's mimetic theory of desire, we want what others want. And without rules and constraints over perhaps the most emotional desire in our life, things can quickly get out of hand.

Put two kids together with a surplus of toys and their desire(s) will inevitably latch onto the same toy, beginning a tug-of-war and mutual cries that 'I wanted it (or had it) first!'[4]

So it seems that monogamy is supported by religion to keep us civilised and restrain us from sliding into all out no-rules competition and violence with each other. As the famous relationship therapist Esther Perel says: *It is the only commandment in the Bible that is repeated twice.*[5]

It is clear that mimetic rivalry is an incubator and accelerator of human violence. Mimetic forces left unchecked by external societal checks would result in contagious spasms of violence.[6]

The upshot of all this is that the need for rules of engagement around sexual rivalry in society is so that the phenomenon of envy and jealousy is *preconscious*. It is a deeply rooted emotion that needs great care and deliberation for couples to consciously venture outside of.

---

3. https://www.wbur.org/modernlove/2019/02/06/marry-husband-winger-rosenthal

4. https://woodybelangia.com/what-is-mimetic-theory/

5. https://www.youtube.com/watch?v=P2AUat93a8Q

6. https://woodybelangia.com/what-is-mimetic-theory/

Even if what a jealous husband claims about his wife (that she sleeps around with other men) is all true, his jealousy is still pathological. —Jacques Lacan, French psychoanalyst (1901-1981)

Insecurity

Perhaps a more emotional reason for limiting our partners freedom is rooted in an unconscious insecurity fear that we are incapable of keeping our partner interested in us.[7] Perhaps we fear that, if we released the emotional collar around our partner's neck, they might not return to us. Would they continue choosing us if they had the option of choosing someone younger, thinner, more attractive, richer, spiritually-evolved or more charismatic?

Insecurity is a very real and fundamental emotion that we can't pretend we don't feel... until we don't. But is there a bridge between the two?

De-legitimising Jealousy

Some people in polyamorous communities have found useful tools to actively de-legitimise jealousy, which requires a significant degree of emotional self-development. One way to do it is choosing to act from our rational mind instead of from our emotionally-conditioned, knee-jerk reactions while, at the same time, *not pretending* we don't feel those emotions.

In those communities it is not uncommon to hear someone who has worked a lot on this topic saying something like, *'Sure! I experience jealousy, but I try not to act from it. I don't believe that my negative emotions are a good reason for my lover not to do what we've agreed would be the most evolved way to proceed. I would rather deal with my emotions and grow through them, than use them to emotionally manipulate my lover into behaving in a certain way.'*

In this way, they acknowledge the emotional reaction but they don't give it power over themselves or the relationship. This requires being honest about feelings whilst keeping them in perspective and thus avoiding a fake, non-jealous persona.[8]

---

7. https://www.psychologytoday.com/us/blog/rediscovering-love/201801/insecurity
8. https://www.psychologytoday.com/us/blog/love-without-limits/201111/polyamory-without-tears

Jealousy Can Be Transcended Through Practice

Jealousy is something that can be transcended, but most people never dare to address the issue because doing so can be intimidating and require huge amounts of personal (and potentially painful) growth. However, the potential reward is as great as the effort it requires.

We covered open relationships in the last chapter but here are a few extra points that relate specifically to jealousy and how to deal with it:

- Jealousy is sometimes bigger in the mind than in reality. When you are ready for it, ask to sit and watch your partner interact with someone, agreeing that you can *'pull the hand break'* at any moment, if it becomes too much. The jealousy spell can be broken and replaced with unconditional love *if* you can manage to stay *really* present in what is actually happening, beyond your thoughts. Can you *be happy they are happy*, and feel the generosity of your most unconditionally-loving side?
- Start with someone you both trust and choose together. Make sure you pick a person of integrity that you *both* feel would not try to steal your partner away from you.
- At first, pick someone who doesn't trigger your fears of inadequacy. Someone you feel confident your partner would not *permanently* prefer over you.
- Slowly, work your way up to more *threatening* lovers. For example, people who are younger, more attractive or more successful than yourself. The upside of this is that you will learn through the *evidence of choice* that your partner is actively choosing you as their long-term partner. There is no bigger compliment or reassurance than being wanted by your partner when they have full permission to play with whoever they want and continually return to you.

Compersion

You will know when you have fully transcended jealousy when you get turned-on by watching your partner being sexual with another person. This feeling of being happy and horny because your partner is experiencing sexual pleasure with someone else, is called *compersion*. It's a feeling of deep empathy for your partner, in which their sexual joy becomes your joy.[9,10]

It might even happen that you become happy to relax watching some Netflix and actually appreciate that someone you trust is *'sharing the work-load'* with you! After all, what could be better than having your partner return home happy, horny and grateful, especially when you didn't have to put in all the physical effort yourself? A win-win-win!

Just because you feel compersion once, doesn't mean you will always feel it. However, when you experience it, you have evidence that it *is* possible. So, the next time jealousy rears its ugly head, you can approach yourself with compassion and curiosity and ask: *'What do I feel insecure about? What needs do I have that aren't being met?'*

But, What If...?

What if your worst fears actually come true and your partner prefers to stay with the new person? If you can look at it purely from an objective, rational mind, doesn't it seem likely that, in the end, you were really not the best match? In that case, everything boils down to the following question: can you be happier by yourself, knowing you aren't compromising by keeping the wrong person around, just because you can't handle being alone? This is another opportunity for growth, so if your growth and personal development is your highest priority, then you really can't lose. But that is a big *'if'*.

If you have checked yourself multiple times but you still feel something is not right with the situation, consider that perhaps your *'spidey senses'* might be tingling for a legitimate reason. Is there something that is not clean in these interactions? Is there a hidden objective in someone? Again, awareness, communication, radical honesty and a high degree of self-ex-ploration will be the tools that should be able to help you accelerate your development in this high-stakes arena.

Photo credit: *Rúben Gál* (https://pixabay.com/users/gallila-photo-695085/), https://pixabay.com/photos/young-girl-jealousy-passion-1349151/

---

9. https://spectrumboutique.com/blog/2019/03/18/ compersion-the-polyamory-hack-to-improve-all-of-your-relationships/

10. https://www.psychologytoday.com/us/blog/the-polyamorists-next-door/201312/ jealousy-and-compersion-multiple-partners-1

23

TANTRA HAS NOTHING TO DO WITH SEX

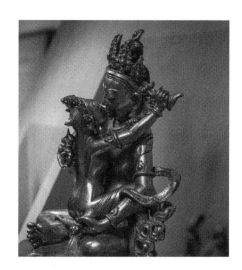

Who Says?

One of the criticisms by the self-appointed *tantra police experts* is that *'tantra is not about sex'*. This usually seems to emanate from those that are heavily inclined towards the more conservative paths that might want to avoid the messy stuff... and yes, sex is messy in more ways than one.

If you read the Tantras themselves, it is obvious that all this [no sex] is nonsense. They are explicit and unambiguous about the central and necessary role of sexual practice in Tantra. Only by Herculean feats of deliberate misinterpretation can they be made to seem to say otherwise. —David Chapman.[1]

In Tantra there is a bigger picture reason for specifically including sex: fixing your sex life can lead to fixing your life in general. If you work things out in one of the most difficult areas of your life you might just find that the same principals work surprisingly well in less volatile domains.

One reason sex is often excluded from tantric practices is that it keeps practices radically embodied, and for that reason it *is* more *intense* and scary. Underlying neuroses, hangups and jealousy issues *will* be exposed, together with any undesirable motives for compulsive sexual impulses.

---

1. https://buddhism-for-vampires.com/tantra-sex-romance-novels

Good tantra should provide useful skills and wisdom to constructively address issues and if done right, there should be a correlating reflection in daily life. Thus the aim of this book is to go beyond just *better sex* and actually change many areas of your life for the better.

Another benefit of including the difficult sexual embodiment practices is that it leaves little chance for the spiritual ego to escape in philosophical back-patting and self-congratulation. But the decision between the sex-exclusive or sex-inclusive path is obviously up to you and I'm certainly not implying that one method is superior over the other.

'This is Not Real Tantra'

Another common misunderstanding flaunted by the *'cultural appropriation police'* is that modern western tantra is not *real* tantra. Fortunately tantra has now entered a new phase of vivid dialogue between East and West, both enriching each other. The beauty of the Western is that we can utilise the best aspects, such as modern science, to update and expand the traditional Eastern Tantric philosophies. In fact, many of the general principles of Tantra have long been found in the West, for example in William Blake and Nietzsche:

The road of excess leads to the palace of wisdom... You never know what is enough until you know what is more than enough. —(1793) William Blake, Proverbs of Hell.[2]

Once hadst thou passions and calledst them evil. But now hast thou only thy virtues: they grew out of thy passions. Thou implantedst thy highest aim into the heart of those passions: then became they thy virtues and joys. And though thou wert of the race of the hot-tempered, or of the voluptuous, or of the fanatical, or the vindictive; All thy passions in the end became virtues, and all thy devils angels. Once hadst thou wild dogs in thy cellar: but they changed at last into birds and charming songstresses. —Friedrich Nietzsche (1844-1900), 'Thus Spake Zarathustra.'[3]

This is not a new debate as the sex/intensity debate has been around for a long time. There are even 2 clear paths in delineating this difference

2. https://www.goodreads.com/quotes/665209-the-road-of-excess-leads-to-the-palace-of-wisdom-you

3. http://www.literaturepage.com/read/thusspakezarathustra-40.html

in Buddhism. The more *calm and controlled* or the more *intense* and *highly provocative.*

Buddhist Framework

In Buddhist philosophical framework there is even terminology outlining those two different schools of practice. The more calm and conservative path (Sutra—renunciation and purification) or the more wild and inclusive path (Tantra—transformation of desire through serving and constructive action):

Sutra recommends that you minimise your exposure to such emotionally provocative situations. It recommends that you develop equanimity to meet them without passion when you cannot avoid them. Tantra recommends that you gradually increase your ability to act effectively in extreme situations, by developing spaciousness and passion together. You can do that relatively safely by deliberately creating intensity, in a controlled situation. There you practice meeting strong feelings with accommodating space. Tantra is extreme because reality is extreme. One way or another, you are going to have to deal with sex, love, loss, conflict, failure, and our good friends 'old age, sickness, and death.' —David Chapman.[4]

In fact one can't practice Tantra without a firm base in Sutra. For example — the tantric non-spasm-orgasm practice is a very real example of Sutric renunciation and makes the practices prescribed in this book less appealing to those who might initially see tantra as an excuse to act out pure hedonism. So although they are quite distinct paths, there is also overlap.

OK. Can we get back to the dick talk now?

Photo credit: *KiraHundeDog* (https://pixabay.com/users/kirahundedog-1347708/), https://pixabay.com/photos/buddha-tantra-stature-shiva-shakti-4642497/

---

4. https://vividness.live/2012/08/05/our-buddhism-goes-to-eleven/

24

STRAIGHT MEN DON'T LIKE DICK

Some Things Can't Be Reversed

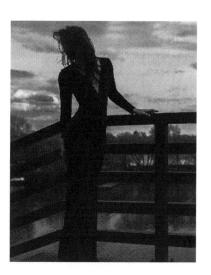

Let's get this straight — liking dick doesn't make you necessarily gay.[1] Come on guys, be honest... Don't you just adore your own dick? If you were a contortionist in *Cirque du Soleil*, wouldn't you use that level of flexibility during your downtime to do some self-pleasuring? If not, do you only watch lesbian porn? Do you avert your eyes from any penises in hetero-sexual porn?

As a gender-fluid person, every time I go out dressed in full femme re-galia, I learn a little more about men's desires and penis fear (or lack there-of). If I'm walking down the street in a very progressive city like London, Amsterdam or Paris, 50% of the men who approach me don't care when they find out that I have a dick under my dress. In fact, there is a substantial segment of the straight male population that actively seeks transgender women.[2] I can't count how many times I've heard the phrase *the perfect woman*, and not just from men. What may surprise you is the huge number of women that hit on trans women.

Thanks to people like Ru Paul and her incredibly successful double-digit

1. https://www.thecut.com/2017/02/how-straight-men-explain-their-same-sex-encounters.html

2. https://www.vice.com/en_us/article/43jzvb/straight-men-recall-the-first-time-they-were-attracted-to-a-trans-woman

seasons of *Drag Race*, gender fluidity is becoming progressively more accepted in society every year. It seems that we are steadily moving towards a growing acceptance of diversity and, as recent modelling trends show, to the point in which androgyny is even becoming a desirable trait.

Charisma is the radiance produced by the interaction of male and female elements in a gifted personality. —Camille Paglia

Country Acceptance Varies

If acceptance of diversity is a true gauge of a country's open-mindedness, perhaps transsexuals should not be coerced, incentivised or railroaded into cutting off their penises if they don't *freely* choose to do so. I've met a significant number of post-operative transgender women who have later regretted cutting off their penises. From that perspective, it seems unfortunate that in some countries, the government will generously pay for sexual reassignment surgery, but *only* if they do the whole shebang, so to speak. Perhaps this sends a clear (but unspoken) message that people should choose one gender or the other and not sit on the fence, implying that the middle-ground is, somehow, an illegitimate 3rd option. Pressure can lead to regrets.[3,4]

Some cultures have a place for people who are neither fully male nor female. In history, trans people have been accepted as a legitimate part of society in some cultures. In Chapter 12 we gave a few examples and here are a few more. Ancient Egyptians seemed to have recognised a third gender.[5] The Zapotec culture accepts people who were born male but behave as females as a third gender referred to as *Muxe*.[6] In Japan, *Kabuki* actors during the Edo period were men who played the role of women both on and off stage. In the Philippines, men who dress and behave like women

3. Djordjevic, Miroslav L., et al. 'Reversal surgery in regretful male-to-female transsexuals after sex reassignment surgery.' *The journal of sexual medicine* 13.6 (2016): 1000-1007.

4. https://www.independent.co.uk/life-style/gender-reversal-surgery-demand-rise-assignment-men-women-trans-a7980416.html

5. Sethe, K. (1926), Die Aechtung feindlicher Fürsten, Völker und Dinge auf altägyptischen Tongefäßscherben des mittleren Reiches, in: *Abhandlungen der Preussischen Akademie der Wissenschaften*, Philosophisch-Historische Klasse (p. 61)

6. Chiñas, B. (1995) Isthmus Zapotec attitudes toward sex and gender anomalies, in Stephen O. Murray (ed.) (1995). *Latin American Male Homosexualities* (pp. 293-302). Albuquerque: University of New Mexico Press.

are considered to be a third gender known as *Bakla*.[7] There are many other examples, but relatively few of them in Western countries, at least until recent times.

The point is that variety is the spice of life and the more options we have to choose from the better. The more accepting and loving a society becomes, the more transsexuals can move out of the shadows of abnormality as a sexual object of perversion, and a creative expression in the diverse spectrum of gender. Not all straight men are dick shy. Just sayin'.

What it will really take to move acceptance to the next level, is for a free-thinking radical A-lister like Keanu Reeves who really doesn't care so much about what people think of him to openly date a transexual. Imagine that. *'I just love the person and that is not changed by what is between her legs... besides, it's really none of your business what we do in the bedroom.'*

Now that's a man! I'm up for it.

Photo credit: *Khusen Rustamov* (https://pixabay.com/users/xusenru-1829710/), https://pixabay.com/photos/long-dress-slim-girl-model-1438140/

---

7. Vonne Patiag, *The Guardian*, Sun 3 Mar 2019. In the Philippines they think about gender differently. We could too, https://www.theguardian.com/world/2019/mar/03/in-the-philippines-they-think-about-gender-differently-we-could-too

25

MOST WOMEN CAN'T SQUIRT

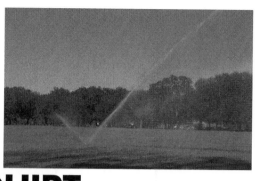

Squirting School

It's a shame that most women don't think they are capable of ejaculating when they orgasm. I've been assured by countless women that the experience of having a powerful, squirting orgasm is vastly different and more satisfying than a clitoral orgasm. It seems like it is not a new phenomenon as Dr Graaf tests to:

The discharge from the female 'prostatae' causes as much pleasure as does that from the male 'prostatae' —Dr Regnier de Graaf (1641 – 1673) Dutch physician and anatomist

Squirting for Everyone!

If you were born with a vagina, chances are that you can squirt. A 1994 study by Stanislav Kratochvil revealed that only about 6% of the Czech women studied were able to ejaculate.[1] In my experience, virtually all women are able to learn how to squirt if they can overcome a couple of hurdles.[2] There are two major factors that often prevent women from being capable of ejaculating. The first one is a lack of knowledge about the technique, and the second is shame. As if women didn't have enough shame around

---

1. https://www.psychologytoday.com/us/blog/all-about-sex/201401/female-ejaculation-what-s-known-and-unknown

2. International sexologist Deborah Sundahl also believes that every woman can squirt. See https://www.salon.com/2015/05/20/the_secret_to_female_ejaculation_how_all_women_can_experience_it_partner/

sex in general, squirting can bring up pee shame as well.

To Pee or Not to Pee?

One of the first questions I hear from women when they learn to squirt is *'Is it pee?'* In 2014, French doctors conducted a study of 7 women capable of ejaculating in large volumes.[3] The liquid they produced during ejaculation was evaluated and found to be mostly urine plus fluid from the female prostate — the Skenes gland. Furthermore, in five out of the seven women, the ejaculated fluid contained prostatic acid phosphatase (PSA), which is also found in male ejaculation and is considered to help sperm motility.[4]

Squirting is not just for the woman's pleasure. Most men seem to enjoy a woman's sexual fountain but it does seem to vary by country and culture. *'Squirt'* became the most searched porn category in Belarus in 2018![5] So, if you are going to learn how to squirt (or if you're going to help your partner learn), then maybe it is time to relax the pee shame and get on with the liquid fireworks. Here are some useful preparations that will make the whole affair far more enjoyable.

Set the Scene

If you were going to paint in your bedroom, you would certainly put down some drop cloths to avoid ruining the floor, right? Well, if you don't properly prepare, you'll end up with a soaking wet bed (and maybe even floor and walls as well!). We have all been trained since our earliest years to avoid having *'accidents'* in bed, so there is usually some conditioning to transcend while learning to squirt. Proper preparation can help relax the mind knowing that a quick and painless clean up follows the pleasure. Towels are fine, but better yet, invest in a waterproof mattress cover to put on the bed, and leave it on under your fitted sheet. Then when *'thunderbirds are go'* you'll be ready for the female version of Viagra... Niagara!

---

3. https://onlinelibrary.wiley.com/doi/epdf/10.1111/jsm.12799?referrer_access_token=t4GbQwAL5-GNarw3eBWZQota6bR2k8jH0KrdpFOxC65memqKNsfjsuAn1r Mecy6id1i_yrDnSYTo9ZQkMjV4cGGeEc_0Rs2SVxW_IlsOGgClyGwYqEwXEJ7h6kof-pz0ZTg9y5VG-6DsTEdWoliTyg%3D%3D

4. https://www.medicalnewstoday.com/articles/323953.php

5. https://www.pornhub.com/insights/2018-year-in-review

Let's Get Started

Now that you have waterproofed your bed, you may still need to do a little work to feel secure about releasing all that liquid that builds up during arousal. For example, a man supporting his female partner on her maiden voyage may need to tell her how sexy he thinks it is to see women ejaculate. He should ideally tell her about it before, during and after as well... at least until she becomes a squirt veteran.

One simple tip is to invite her to pee before you start. When a woman empties her bladder beforehand, it becomes easier for her to understand that this is not just like urinating in the bed. Also, the ejaculated liquid will be more clear and have less odour than if she didn't.[6,7,8]

Fingering

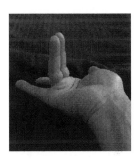

Let's assume you have already de-armoured the G-spot as taught in earlier chapters... otherwise there will be pain instead of pleasure. There is a different use of the fingers in this type of orgasm. Instead of finger banging in and out style, you want to make tiny circular motions using your fingertips like a mini *Karate Kid* internally doing the *wax on, wax off* thang.

Have a look at the photo here to get the correct finger position of your submersible karate guy. Hold your hand palm facing up and you raise the middle two fingers. Hold them rigidly perpendicular to your palm like a tree trunk. You now have the correct finger position.

To begin the stimulation, start by placing just the middle finger up towards the G-spot and move it in a gentle circular motion against the ridges of the G-spot. These ridges feel like the ridges on the roof of your mouth. This phase is called *polishing the mirror*. Keep doing this until you feel the G-spot swell into the size of an almond. Keep communicating and ask her how it feels. If it feels pleasurable accompanied by a *'I need to pee'*

---

6. Salama, Samuel, et al. 'Nature and origin of 'squirting' in female sexuality.' *The journal of sexual medicine* 12.3 (2015): 661-666.

7. https://www.bbc.co.uk/bbcthree/article/544c5686-e3bc-4ac2-b4ca-f91eccefe441

8. https://www.sciencealert.com/where-female-ejaculation-comes-from-and-what-it-s-made-of

sensation, then you know you are on the right track.

The second part of this process is much more forceful, so use the stronger two-finger method (as in the photo) and keep checking with her how it feels so you don't hurt her. With the middle two fingers in the vagina, press them down towards the anus quite strongly. Then, move those two rigid fingers upwards towards the G-spot and squish it against the pubic bone.[9] Use the back of your fingers to press towards her anus, then you pull up to squish her G-spot with the front of your straight fingers. Don't let the tree trunk loose its rigidity. Remember to keep asking her how it feels. If she says 'good', then you can experiment even a little harder. As long as you don't hurt her, you will be surprised by how strongly you can continue with these up-and-down strokes. You will know you are doing it correctly when you hear juicy slurping sounds on the downstroke as suction is produced between the palm of your hand and the *labia majora*.

You've probably never used your hand in this way before, so you might get tired surprisingly quickly. There are a couple of things that you can do. You can support the hand that's doing all the work by grabbing your wrist with your free hand and aid the up-and-down working hand. You can also switch arms to give yourself a break. A little trick is to *start* with your non-dominant hand, so by the time she is ready for full-power, you can swap to your dominant hand. Over time, you will learn to read her body and become able to help her ejaculate within a couple of minutes, or even seconds!

There are two different ways in which women can ejaculate, softly or forcibly. The technique explained above is quite forceful and it's a useful starting point on this path and far easier to learn. The negative part is that it can drop a woman's sexual energy, somewhat. This is a little similar to how men lose energy after ejaculation. The more difficult *soft ejaculation* method only really occurs with womb orgasms but doesn't lead to a drop in energy for the woman. It is a totally different method that we will cover in the chapter dedicated to womb orgasm.

Photo 1 credit:
Runawayfromzombies (https://pixabay.com/users/runawayfromzombies-4313703/), https://pixabay.com/photos/sprinkler-park-rainbow-grass-lawn-1993799/
Photo 2 credit: *Alexa Vartman*

---

9. https://www.healthline.com/health/g-spot-in-women

26

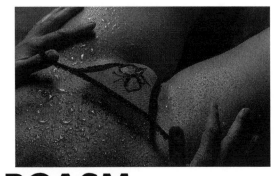

THE
CERVIX
CAN'T ORGASM
The Deep Pleasure Button

Many people may find it surprising that cervical stimulation can lead to orgasm.[1] Even women who are sexually open may balk at the idea of the cervix as a pleasure centre. But in fact, the cervix contains a huge number of nerve endings from the *hypogastric*, *pelvic* and *vagus* nerves. These three nerves perform feedback to the brain during sexual stimulation which can act as a doorway to intense pleasurable cervical orgasms. Even women with spinal cord injury have reported that they can cervically orgasm and this has been attributed to the vagus nerve:

> *Since most of those nerves are associated with the spinal cord, it would stand to reason that a person with a severed spinal cord wouldn't be able to have an orgasm. And for a very long time, that's what people with these types of injuries were told. However, recent studies show that people with spinal cord injuries—even paraplegics—can reach orgasm. Dr. Barry Komisaruk and Dr. Beverly Whipple of Rutgers University conducted a study on women with severed spinal cords in 2004. They discovered that these women could feel stimulation of their cervixes and even reach orgasm, although there was no way their brain could be receiving information from the hypogastric or pelvic nerves. How was this possible? An MRI scan of the women's brains showed that the region corresponding to signals from the vagus nerve was active. Because the vagus bypasses the spinal cord, the women were still able to feel*

---

1. https://www.glamour.com/story/
   how-to-have-a-cervical-orgasm-according-to-a-neuroscientist

cervical stimulation. —Shanna Freeman, *HowStuffWorks.*[2]

However, as I mentioned earlier in the section about vaginal de-armouring in chapter 9, chances are that sexually experienced women are unconsciously experts at wiggling their hips to one side to avoid painful thrusts of the penis against their cervix.[3,4] Dodging their partner's incoming member has probably become second-nature, to avoid getting hurt. Instead of perpetually dodging the bullet, wouldn't it be more fun if we could change the game from *'hide and seek'* to pleasurable *'smash and grab'*?

If you are an office worker, then you experience that tense shoulders are not an uncommon side-effect of sitting for hours at a computer. Although you haven't been intentionally working out those shoulder muscles, they may feel like you have. This is because the tensions of the day often take up residence between your shoulder blades. If you get a deep-tissue massage, it might hurt at first, but as the massage therapist presses and pounds those sore muscles, they start to relax.

Similarly, women seem to store tension and stress in the cervix.[5,6] The first step towards being able to experience pleasure in the cervix is to remove that tension. As we discussed in Chapter 9, the cervix can be de-armoured. Women generally only need to have their vaginas de-armoured one time, but the cervix is another story altogether. Women seem to slowly accumulate tension in the cervix and they can benefit from being de-armoured before sex... most naturally, with the penis.

How to Soften the Cervix

Let's recap the cervix de-armouring process we described in Chapter 9, but this time, rather than using the finger method which is the preferred method for the first major de-armouring, we will go into more detail on how to use the penis to do the regular shorter maintenance.

At the start of sex, once you have penetrated her and checked for pain with the penis, press and hold the head of your penis against her cervix

2. https://health.howstuffworks.com/sexual-health/sexuality/brain-during-orgasm1.htm

3. https://www.bustle.com/articles/119634-what-its-like-to-have-a-bruised-cervix-the-sex-injury-that-no-one-talks-about

4. https://www.healthywomen.org/content/article/could-you-have-bruised-cervix

5. https://www.calmclinic.com/anxiety/symptoms/vaginal-discomfort

6. https://pelvicpainhelp.com/reducing-anxiety-heal-pelvic-pain/

and ask her how that feels. Just like the massage therapist needs feedback to learn how much pressure to use, the male partner needs to know how hard to press against the cervix. Too little, and the cervix will not soften, too hard and she won't come back for more. If she feels no pain, then press the penis in progressively harder until you hear something along the lines of 'Ouch... *mother fucker... yes, there!'* Then, press and hold for a minute or so until the pain subsides.

If you want a more graphic first-hand description of what it feels like for the man to do this process, skip to the last few chapters of this book.

What if I Lose My Erection?

Cervical de-armouring is more like a medical procedure than fun, so, as the man, you will undoubtedly find yourself becoming soft in the process.[7] Take a 30-second break and create a little friction and pleasure to regain your lost wood. Once you stop pressing against the cervix, the pain will subside, and you can enjoy for a few moments but, sooner or later, the process needs to be completed by pressing the head of your penis hard against the cervix.

Tilt her hips upwards towards you with your hands to make the cervix more vulnerable, then use your penis to press against the pointy part of the cervix and pay attention to her breath. If you notice that she is holding her breath, it is probably because you hit the bullseye. You may even be able to feel where the cervix is with your penis.

Keep pressing until the cervix has *virtually* no pain and only slight discomfort, then slow, rhythmic bumps against the cervix will overwhelm the slight discomfort with pleasure. Keep asking for feedback and get progressively harder, while you follow her verbal and bodily cues.

How to Deal with a Tough Façade

Many women have been trained to avoid showing pain in bed. They may have the notion that women who experience pain during sex are uptight,

---

7. No judgment against sadists, some of my best friends are sadists.

unrelaxed or unsexy.[8,9] This is yet another reason why it is important to keep communicating. Remember, this experience is not just physical, it's also emotional, mental, and perhaps even a little spiritual.

The tension will not leave the cervix unless the woman can become vulnerable and express her pain through her mouth. The *tough woman* routine is the exact opposite of what will help dissipate the tension. It takes a lot of bravery to be purposefully and consciously weak. Luckily, a deep vulnerability can allow these recently created layers of the cervix pain to release in a minute or two.

No More Physical Pain. Now What?

Sorry ladies, this is just level one. We're peeling an onion here. Once the outer level of pain has been removed, we still need to release the final deeper tension. The next step is for the man to place the woman's ankles over his shoulders to gain maximum exposure to the cervix. This step will take out the last remaining tension accumulated right in the centre of the opening. This is an incredibly vulnerable position, so be fully present and mindful of every movement, and also reassure her that she is in charge of the process and the level of pressure you use.

Press, cry, release, repeat.

Once the cervix has no pain, you can test it by bumping your cock against it with a little movement. Very short strokes, more like a jab. Just keep checking if there is any pain. If the answer is *'No, it feels really nice!'* then you can start to enjoy and play more with this new-found toy. You might both be surprised just how pleasurable it feels when you pound a really soft and rubbery cervix.[10,11]

A word of advice to guys: Be careful as she is writhing around on the end of your dick. This is a lot of horny energy to conduct for any man.

---

8. Stockman, J. A. 'Why Do Young Women Continue to Have Sexual Intercourse Despite Pain? Elmerstig E, Wijma B, Berterö C (Linköping Univ, Sweden; et al) J Adolesc Health 43: 357-363, 2008.' *Year Book of Pediatrics* 2010 (2010): 9-11.

9. Stout, Madison E., Samantha M. Meints, and Adam T. Hirsh. 'Loneliness Mediates the Relationship Between Pain During Intercourse and Depressive Symptoms Among Young Women.' *Archives of sexual behavior* 47.6 (2018): 1687-1696.

10. https://www.sexcoaching.com/sexual-pleasure/cervical-orgasm/

11. https://www.refinery29.com/en-us/what-is-a-cervical-orgasm-tips

You will probably have to put the brakes on fairly frequently at the start until you get really good at moving that cervix-sex electricity through your spasm reflex zone towards your tailbone. Over time it will become second nature and *friction-only* sex will become rather unappealing and more like beginners sex.

Go, team! You have just helped her to experience one of the deepest orgasms and releases a woman can have.[12,13] She will feel the effects of this highly-pleasurable experience for quite some time afterwards. A nice consequence for the provider is that you can rest assured that you have set a pretty high bar. When facilitating cervical orgasms becomes part of your sexual toolbox, you're definitely bringing some serious sex-skills to the bedroom and your A-game will be hard to match.

Photo credit: *Poszarobert* (https://pixabay.com/users/poszarobert-7518426/?tab=about), https://pixabay.com/photos/a-people-naked-girl-adult-nude-3049572/

12. https://www.vice.com/en_us/article/434wxb/
this-is-how-to-hit-the-other-g-spot-the-a-spot

13. https://www.cosmopolitan.com/sex-love/advice/a6896/cervical-orgasm-guide/

27

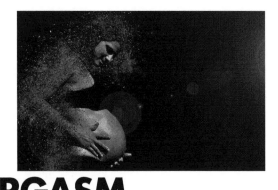

THE WOMB CAN'T ORGASM
Training for Pain-Free Childbirth

Most people don't realise that there are 7 different orgasms a woman can have through 4 unique nerve pathways.

We recognise four different nerve pathways that carry sensory signals from the vagina, cervix, clitoris and uterus, and they all can contribute to orgasms. That's a new recognition. —Barry Komisaruk

The uterus can also deeply orgasm, and more intensely than the clitoris, G-spot, anal or even cervical orgasm... and for many minutes longer. There are also very specific physical symptoms that happen when the womb orgasms, which distinguish it from the other tantric orgasms. Here are some reports from several women that have experienced this rare orgasm:

This orgasm is like an explosion from deep within.

I was more out of control than I have ever been, sexually.

It was a spiritually-healing experience.

All I could do was moan and growl, and then, afterwards, I cried because of the intensity of the release.

I woke up orgasming the day after.

Days later, I would still have spontaneous orgasms, like the aftershocks of an intense earthquake.

I had a pervasive feeling of peace and deep satisfaction that lasted for days.

To experience this deepest, tantric orgasm, the woman does not need to do more than be able to orgasm on the cervix, as explained in the previous chapter. For the man, there are a couple of extra skills required.

How Do You Give a Womb Orgasm?

Initiating a woman's very first womb orgasm is pretty much up to the skills of a tantric man, and it might take months or years for him to be able to master this practice. Physically, the man will need to have his genitals and anus de-armoured, and his spine sexually-activated, but that is just the beginning. To produce a womb orgasm, the man must be able to produce sexual energy inside the woman's vagina without using friction. This is difficult to describe in words, but the basic concept is that you practise *'edging'* and surfing at 99% to the point of orgasm, with less and less friction, until you can surf that edge without any movement.[1] I don't know any other way to describe that physical sensation without putting you inside my body, but practising to *'edge'* while masturbating tantrically (as described in this book), is an essential preparation towards it. As you become more sensitive to feeling the subtle sexual energy currents, simply resting the head of the penis against the cervix will produce a really pleasant feeling of *'I'm almost about to cum'*.[2] That tingling sensation will probably make you suddenly feel the need to *'back away'* from the cervix, or it will overwhelm you. Practise holding at 99% of the point of no return (without requiring any movement to create that pleasure) for longer and longer, until you can stay there indefinitely. If you do this right, this will make the woman go crazy in horniness... And here lies the problem. The hornier she becomes, the more difficult it will be to conduct her full sexual force. It's quite something!

If I haven't had sex for many months (which is all too common these days), I notice that I lose my practice and have to get her to *dial it down* until I can acclimatise myself again. Perhaps she needs to be quieter and less vocal, no hip bucking and definitely no squeezing of the vagina. If she bucks her hips, it becomes almost impossible to control your sensations. I guess this is similar to walking down an unseen step at night when your brain doesn't expect the sudden drop. Making intentional movements when your brain knows what to expect greatly decreases sensation, kind

---

1. https://www.kinkly.com/definition/1162/orgasm-control

2. https://melmagazine.com/en-us/story/
    my-college-girlfriend-thought-the-mormon-dick-soak-would-preserve-her-virginity

of like the way tickling yourself doesn't work so well.[3]

If I have had sex recently but had an orgasm by mistake, it becomes *more* difficult to produce this buzzing feeling in the penis. Contrary to popular belief, it is *more* difficult to not go over the edge for about 2 weeks after ejaculating. The reason is that although you might be less horny, the longer you don't ejaculate the further away that spasm reflex gets. One explanation might be that if you've used that neural pathway recently, the habit can quickly return.

Once you can rest your tingling, tantric penis against the cervix for a long time, you can move to the following step. Feeling the tingling sensation in the penis, add friction and movement. Start with gentle, slow, unexpected prods against the cervix. If she is fully de-armoured, this will make her go crazy, but if not, she will feel some pain there, and you will need to de-armour her cervix by pressing hard against it with your penis as described in the last chapter. Only proceed to the phase of bumping against the cervix when *all* the pain has gone.

Over time (both long-term and per session), you will be able to handle more and more stimulation. Eventually, you will be capable of pounding her cervix as hard as she is screaming for it, and for as long as needed to produce the womb orgasm. When you witness a woman in full sexual rapture, you will understand first-hand why tantric tradition claims that women are more sexually wild than men! This is the point where the value of sexual control is at its highest. Many women report that they can't fully let go of their sexual energy because that will push the man over the point of no return, so they learn to restrain themselves.

Eventually, she will be begging you to really go to town on her via the cervix. To bring the intensity required, you have to kill the little boy inside of you and tap into your anger to transform it into manly service. *'Rage against the cervix'* for the sake of your partner. She will be out of her mind, in absolute rapture, in her deepest surrender and writhing around on the end of your penis. Once her cervix trusts the penis and has been able to fully let go, this will provide an energetic pathway to the womb.[4,5]

3. https://www.scientificamerican.com/article/why-cant-a-person-tickle/

4. https://www.kinkly.com/seven-sexy-facts-to-help-you-reach-cervical-climax/2/17428

5. https://www.shape.com/lifestyle/sex-and-love/cervical-orgasms

Divine Slut Mode

When the womb orgasms, it is like an earthquake in the deepest part of the body, with obvious signs that cannot be faked. The vagina will involuntarily bellow air in-and-out as it opens like a balloon and then contracts forcibly, expelling air. Oftentimes, this will be accompanied by her frequent, slow and steady ejaculation, something I call *'oiling the tools'*. I like to rapidly end the pounding by counting backwards from 10 to 0 to give her adequate warning that the session is about to stop, and then pull out quickly and watch her body twist and contort in spontaneous temple-dancing like movements, called *'mudras'*. The whole affair is beyond intense. Her eyes may even appear different, as though she has shifted into a different being. That's one of many benefits of the womb orgasm. It is the most powerful way to reach transcendence of the Matrix without having to use drugs.

Sometimes, strange physiological signs can appear after the womb orgasm. She may cry in gratitude, feeling extreme, open-hearted love for the Universe and everything in it. Unashamed and having revealed her deepest sexuality, she may look 10 years younger and even strangely resemble some sort of tantric goddess. It's certainly the most beautiful thing I have ever seen.

The womb orgasm is good preparation if she ever decides to have children. Womb orgasm sex is tantrically similar to the pain-free, orgasmic birth. An experience that does not create trauma for the infant.[6] This may allow the child to be born without medical intervention, and in overflowing rapture. A nice birthday song to be sure.

We will cover the orgasmic birth in more detail in the last chapter.

Photo credit: *Efes Kitap* (https://pixabay.com/users/efes-18331/),
https://pixabay.com/photos/woman-pregnant-baby-belly-belly-1922353/

---

6. https://www.glamour.com/story/whats-it-actually-like-to-have-an-orgasmic-birth

28

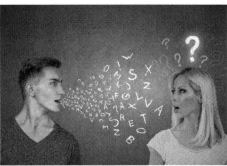

WE SPEAK THE SAME LANGUAGE

Mars Calling Venus

Without emotional trust between you, it's unlikely that she will be able to really let go and relax into deeper tantric orgasms. Trust has to be earned. Have you proven over time that you are not a greedy man just using her? Have you shown that you have a high degree of empathy and aren't going to hurt her? Have you displayed the skills to guide her to relax fully?

Having said that, there are times when even the perfect man would not be good enough. As you practise this deepest form of lovemaking, you may hit a deep layer of emotional resistance in your partner, rooted in the distrust of being directed by a man.[1] Unless the woman was born on a different planet, it's more than likely she's had her heart torn out and stepped on by men who used her body for sex and then carelessly dumped her, in their relentless hunt of the next conquest.[2]

Sometimes in your relationship, she won't even be aware of her resistance or distrust. Perhaps, this lies beyond her personally, as she taps into the collective tension between the genders. Regardless of the reason, expect that sometimes you will receive strange messages uttered in the incomprehensible feminine dialect that will make no sense to your masculine mind.[3] The verbal curve balls she throws in the heat of an argument might

1. https://positivepsychology.com/build-trust/
2. https://www.businessinsider.com/signs-your-old-relationships-are-affecting-your-current-one-2018-6#3-you-have-hangups-around-physical-intimacy-3
3. https://psychcentral.com/blog/6-ways-men-and-women-communicate-differently/

seem to make linguistic sense, but in practice, your masculine, solution-focused mind is ill-equipped to find any actionable content. Sometimes, these cryptic messages are genuine longings, disguised by an inability to *spell it out* in *'guy talk'*. Other times, it may be a cunning way to make a man feel insecure. Thus we need an emotional Babel fish to bridge the gap.

The Classics

Feminine: *'I can't feel your heart!'*

Masculine translation: Often, this means that you are not sweet, kind, romantic or gentle enough to her. Try to feel a loving emotion when you are looking, touching or holding her. In other cases, she might be longing for a more tantric, yogic, energy connection between your hearts. It can be very difficult to know how to address this without some training and practice.

For most women, the language of conversation is primarily a language of rapport: a way of establishing connections and negotiating relationships. —Deborah Tannen, professor of linguistics, Georgetown University, Washington, D.C.

A useful tool to get connected energetically is to imagine opening the right side of your chest (as if a surgeon were using velvet-covered rib-spreaders on you) while feeling a pure form of love and care for her. If you need a life-hack cheat, start the process remembering how you feel with your kids, friends or puppies when you're in one of those *'Hallmark moments'*. Imagine un-contracting the feeling of any perceivable constriction in the right side of your chest and pushing out that *'loving everything'* feeling into the right side of her chest (her energetic heart). I know this all sounds a bit weird, but try it randomly, and see if she notices. You can even try this the next time you are cuddling, and ask her if she feels something out of the ordinary is happening between you. If she says she feels a warm feeling in her heart, jackpot! You might be surprised how much women can tune into that kind of stuff.

Other times she may use this line to simply confuse/outgun you in an area that she has superiority—the realm of feelings. It takes a lot of experience and practice to know the difference between these three uses of the same sentence. Understanding what she is *actually* intending is the key to unlock this feminine *koan* (riddle).

Feminine: *'Be present with me!'*

Masculine translation: Besides not doing two things at once when you are with her, she is probably asking you not to think of something (or someone) else when you are listening to her, touching her or having sex with her.[4]

Feminine: *'Don't be so greedy!'*

Masculine translation: Don't go in with any plans about what you are going to do next with her if those plans involve moving things quickly towards the genitals and orgasm.[5]

Feminine: *'Don't be needy!'*

Masculine translation: Express what you want without being attached to the outcome. Don't be too concerned with getting approval from her. Don't compromise too often and do what feels wrong to you just to please her or to avoid drama.

Feminine: *'Feel me!'*

Masculine translation: She wants you to up your empathic skills and know for yourself what she feels inside her body, mind and emotions without having to tell you. I know it sounds impossible, but it gets easier the more you practise tantric sex. Especially if you spend time in your feminine mode, as described in this book.

Feminine: *'I don't know.'*

Masculine translation: Sometimes, she does know, but she is tired of being in her masculine mode and making the decisions for both of you. She may be asking you to take over the reins and *'man up'* and make some damn decisions! At the same time, she doesn't want you to become selfish and just do what you want. Most likely, she wants you to take her into account by looking at her subtle, body and facial expression in response to her feelings.[6]

---

4. https://www.psychologytoday.com/us/blog/insight-therapy/201502/why-we-cant-stay-focused-during-sex-and-why-it-matters

5. https://www.gq.com/story/esther-perel-what-men-get-wrong-about-sex

6. https://www.bustle.com/articles/167470-9-ways-to-be-more-empathetic-to-your-partner-feel-more-connected-according-to-experts

Feminine: *'Why can't you be more masculine!'*

Masculine translation: We had a whole chapter on this before, and I highly recommend the book *'No more Mr Nice Guy'* for a great read on how to further decipher this cryptic message.[7]

Photo credit: *Pathdoc* (https://www.shutterstock.com/g/pathdoc), https://www.shutterstock.com/image-photo/language-barrier-concept-handsome-man-talking-754147192

---

7. https://www.drglover.com/no-more-mr-nice-guy/the-book.html

29

WOMEN DON'T LIKE DIRTY TALK

It all depends...

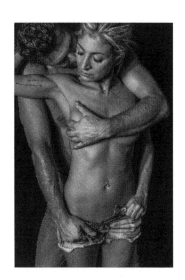

Most super-nice and super-caring men are super bad at dirty-talk. I certainly was a complete moron when it came to the darker verbal repertoire at the start of my tantric training. I thought it sounded like some macho shit, highly disrespectful to women. The type of talk I should help stamp out by being a poster-child for caring and respectful guys everywhere. It was quite a shock to find that *'sweet-boy mode'* wasn't always received as sexy or booty-enticing.[1]

It all seems to hinge on two things: timing and intention. She may rightfully find dirty talk derogatory on the street or when a selfish man objectifies and belittles her. However, in the right situation, it can be a whole other story.[2] Dirty talk does not need to be demeaning, as long as it's done with the right intent, trust, and based on respect.[3] In fact, I am surprised at how the feminine may actually crave the dark verbal arts when done in the right way, with the right person and at the right time.[4]

This can be a difficult conditioning to get over, especially in these hyper-sensitive gender-war times. One of the hidden costs of the *#metoo*

1. https://observer.com/2014/03/ive-got-a-friend-why-are-bad-boys-the-best-in-bed/

2. https://www.refinery29.com/en-us/30-and-single-woman-catcalling

3. https://www.bustle.com/articles/62007-8-reasons-talking-dirty-in-bed-is-good-for-your-relationship

4. https://www.medicaldaily.com/science-dirty-talk-and-why-it-increases-sexual-pleasure-349854

movement is the general lack of confident, assertive men. And, who ends up paying the price for that ultimately? Many women report they lose attraction for banal men that can't convey a wide range of verbal sexual expression. It's a sad fact to see that what started out as a needed and well-intentioned movement, now seems to be (unintentionally) widening the gap between the sexes... or even resulting in over-cautious, neutered males. When rightfully justified censorship of sexist speech in the office creates a bland and politically correct sterile environment in the bedroom, we have probably gone too far. Both sexes lose in this equation. For women, here's why this happens:

While men are generally more visual and tend to respond more to visual stimulation... women, on the other hand, are generally more stimulated by auditory stimuli, and thus usually need more verbal cues than men.[5] This means that the monotonous *'hump, grunt and moan'* soundtrack chiming in her ear might just not do it for her! While sexy moaning can be quite enjoyable, a bit more variety and storyline may be needed to counteract the one playing in her head. She may be listening to the usual feminine soundtrack of not being beautiful, compared to some other woman...[6] or her mother labelling her as *'porky'* or *'too slutty'* when she was sixteen. Good luck countering that with the regular, heavy breathing in her ear! This is where a more creative, darker and more scintillating repartee comes into play.

Dirty Talk: What to Say?

The first time Mr Nice ventures into the darker arts of *'fuck-talk'*, he might be wise to survey the landscape and do some research. Talk about it beforehand. Ask if she wants to try out some new verbal variations. If she agrees, next time you are getting it on, try saying something naughty and see how she responds. If you need a place to start, just describe what you are doing to her and how you feel about it.[7] Follow the direction of her horniness and test what works and what doesn't. You can tell her what you plan to do to her before you actually do it, and test out different scenarios

---

5. https://www.nature.com/articles/ijir201247

6. https://www.psychologytoday.com/us/blog/married-and-still-doing-it/201812/is-body-image-affecting-your-sex-life

7. https://www.huffpost.com/entry/how-to-talk-dirty_l_5cd0c71fe4b0548b735e9062

to see how her body reacts. For example, you can say, *'I'm going to take you in the bedroom now and enjoy that hot little body of yours,'* and see how she responds.

Disturbingly (and shocking to the nice guy), many women enjoy quite graphic fuck-talk. *'Damn your ass looks great in those jeans!'* might sound callous to our conditioned sensibilities, but to some women, from the right guy, in the right moment, might be music to her ears. Feel what happens to her body language when you say that. Does she look at you more sexually, or does she look like she is going to run out of the bedroom in tears? Either response is actually useful from a learning perspective. The most useless response is *indifference*. At least, if she laughs at you, you know you can cross that sentence off your list and test another.[8]

Don't stop as soon as something works (or doesn't). Keep the dirty-talk pattern going. Meet her where she is sexually at that moment by using your words. Initially, she may need some encouragement to let go and embrace her slutty-side, but once she has let go into slut mode, you might be shocked at what can actually work for her.

Initially, get her to help you learn by continuing to respond both positively and negatively so you can navigate more easily. Even to the point of asking her to exaggerate her responses in the learning stage, so you get clear signals.

Not Too Many Questions

One of the most common mistakes men make is asking too many questions, too often. The reason you don't want to do that is you don't want to come across as an insecure little boy, asking mommy's approval for everything you do. *Insecurity and neediness is the #1 turn off for women...* as is trying to be too willing to cater to her every whim.

She might say she likes nice guys... and certainly, you require to have kindness as your core foundation, but being able to overlay that with the guy that is *totally confessed with his desire of her but does not NEED her to be happy, IS a major component of a sexy man*. If you don't believe me, survey a bunch of emotionally-healthy women and see for yourself.

If you still feel at a loss after these explanations, you could check out

---

8. https://www.elitedaily.com/p/telling-your-partner-you-want-them-to-talk-dirty-to-you-is-so-much-easier-than-you-think-17858977

The New Tantra's online video courses. They feature in-depth explanations of basic tantric sexual skills from TNT workshop facilitators and bodyworkers followed by graphic demonstrations. In one of these videos you will find a step-by-step tutorial and demonstration on fuck talk.[9]

Photo credit: *Andrea Altini* (https://pixabay.com/users/andreaaltini-14485571/), https://pixabay.com/photos/boudoir-sexy-woman-girl-attractive-4669610/

---

9. https://courses.thenewtantra.com/

30
ENERGY SEX IS A MYTH

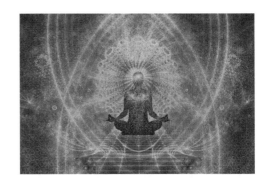

Beyond Friction-Only Sex

The concept of energy sex has nothing to do with energy of the scientific kind. We're not talking about the $E=mc^2$ kind of energy... we're talking about horniness that you can feel mirroring between two people when they are intimate with each other. People practising tantra may notice they become aware of new and subtle forms of sexual connection once the more rudimentary aspects of regular sex are transcended. There are some aspects of energy control that still seem to baffle most areas of science.

Stories of g-tummo meditators mysteriously able to dry wet sheets wrapped around their naked bodies during a frigid Himalayan ceremony have intrigued scholars and laypersons alike for a century. [...] Overall, the results suggest that specific aspects of the g-tummo technique might help non-meditators learn how to regulate their body temperature, which has implications for improving health and regulating cognitive performance. —Kozhevnikov M, Elliott J, Shephard J, Gramann K (2013) Neurocognitive and Somatic Components of Temperature Increases during g-Tummo Meditation.[1]

The meditation mentioned above can also induce extreme orgasmic bliss using breathing and visualisation of a body made of fire. This stuff really

---

1. Kozhevnikov M, Elliott J, Shephard J, Gramann K (2013) *Neurocognitive and Somatic Components of Temperature Increases during g-Tummo Meditation: Legend and Reality.* PLoS ONE 8(3): e58244. https://doi.org/10.1371/journal.pone.0058244

works, surprisingly enough! Energy sex is a core aspect of tantric sex.[2] In tantric lore, you aren't considered a real tantric master unless you can give a woman a full-body orgasm from across the room. Obviously, I cannot demonstrate such a thing in a book, but I have many eyewitnesses from workshops. While you may not be able to make her orgasm with no hands (just yet), developing the ability to consciously move sexual energy is a game-changer, and one of the main differentiating factors to regular sex. Without this, you're eating hot dogs at the kiddie table instead of dining on filet mignon with the adults. No amount of ketchup is going to turn processed pig anuses into steak! There is a whole other world based on the conscious movement of sexual energy, so why not start experimenting and see where it takes you?[3]

An Easier Way to Start Being Sexual

Energy sex is one way you can start to get to know someone in a sexual way without all the risks and baggage that are associated with swapping bodily fluids.[4] It's kind of like kissing first to see if there is a spark. It's safer and doesn't seem to carry the same emotional charge (and mess) as sex with ejaculation.

How to Do Energy Sex?

Let's use a lesbian strap-on scenario to explore what having energy sex can be like... because I assume most people would like to experience lesbian sex, right? To do this, ladies, strap it on and imagine your clitoris is growing into the shape of the attached dildo. Imagine it is an extension of yourself, and slowly slide into your partner. Many women report that when they do this, they feel more as if they had a real cock. Even more interesting, though, some receivers often feel more aliveness or energy in the dildo.[5]

A word of warning, ladies. As you focus your attention on your new, extended clitoris, you might find it is quite easy to become overexcited

---

2. https://www.meetmindful.com/tantric-sex-demystified/

3. https://www.huffpost.com/entry/spiritual-sex-the-art-of_b_261488

4. https://www.psychologytoday.com/us/blog/insight-therapy/201512/stis-risky-scary-or-just-stigmatized

5. Lotney, K. (2000) *The Ultimate Guide to Strap-On Sex: A Complete Resource for Women and Men* (p. 142)

and reach a peak orgasm through the pudendal nerve. You will need to learn how to control your pegging sexual energy, just as a man with a penis needs to. Anus de-armouring, having an activated spine and dissipating your horny energy away from your genitals by slowing down and moving the energy along your perineum, towards your spine, are some useful masculine tools women can adopt if they like to 'top'. I know it may seem implausible, but over time you might experience that your partner can even notice where in their body you place your attention.

Is Energy Sex Real?

For the doubting Thomases out there, here's a more solid example. An experienced tantra practitioner I know was hit from behind on his motor-cycle by a car while sitting stationary in a Dutch traffic jam. His spine was severed at the waist, and he became a paraplegic. He can't feel anything in his penis, and yet he can still get an erection and have sex.[6,7] When I asked him how he does this, he says that he can still sense sexual energy moving in his body, even without the nerves attached, but doubts whether he would have been able to do this without his tantric training.[8,9] He has certainly been an inspiration to me and opened my mind about what's possible with tantra, beyond typical, regularly-agreed conventions.

Photo credit: *Okan Caliskan* (https://pixabay.com/users/activedia-665768/), https://pixabay.com/illustrations/meditation-spiritual-yoga-1384758/

6. Hess, Marika J., and Sigmund Hough. 'Impact of spinal cord injury on sexuality: broad-based clinical practice intervention and practical application.' *The journal of spinal cord medicine* 35.4 (2012): 211-218.

7. https://craighospital.org/resources/sexual-function-for-men-after-spinal-cord-injury

8. https://www.self.com/story/this-is-what-its-like-to-have-sex-as-a-quadriplegic

9. https://medicalxpress.com/news/2009-09-vaginal-orgasm.html

31

ANAL SEX IS A PAIN IN THE ASS

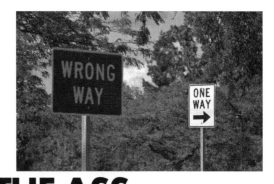

Wrong Technique

Readers of *Georgia Straight*, a leftist magazine based out of the fairly-liberal city of Vancouver, Canada, didn't seem so excited about ass-play. In 2011, the magazine conducted a reader sex survey and asked, amongst other things, *'Have you ever put anything up your ass?'*[1] The response was pretty low, compared to the answers I receive in Europe, but I guess that's to be expected.

- Females who replied *'yes'* = 49.4%.
- Males who replied with a *'yes'* = 28.6% .

Those figures seem rather interesting for a couple of reasons:

1. The figure for men is not insignificant.

2. Women are much higher. Apart from the prostate, men and women have the same physiology, so it probably feels similar to both sexes. It would seem those statistics back up the common belief that women have less shame around anal sex than men. This has probably something to do with *'gay shame'*, which women don't have.

---

1. https://www.straight.com/life/2011-sex-survey-have-you-ever

Does It Have to Hurt?

It's easy to get stuck on the first impression, especially if you tried it once, and it was unpleasant.[2] It seems the ass has a memory like an elephant. Many women report that they have had a negative experience the first time they were penetrated anally.[3] Sometimes, men are not careful about the whole affair. With everything being so slippery down there, they might take an accidental backroad detour and jam his cock into her un-expecting and ill-prepared bum, using the same force he was driving the regular route. (If you aren't wincing or clenching reading this, then you might want to check you have a pulse).

Not only is this painful, but if the next pump is back into her vagina, it can cause a pretty bad urinary tract infection or bacterial vaginosis...[4] which will result in more and longer-lasting pain.

However, it doesn't have to be like this. Anal sex can also be very horny, fun and pain-free.[5] In order to be good at anal sex, the penetrator needs to have empathy with the person being penetrated. Being good at vaginal sex does not necessarily translate into being good at anal sex. The two orifices are quite different in how they need to be approached, as there are different techniques to facilitate pleasure through anal penetration, which we shall cover in more detail here and in other chapters.

For women who wish to experience anal sex for the first time, I have a piece of strong advice... *never allow a man to penetrate your ass if he has not had the experience done well on himself.* While bad vaginal sex is just boring, bad anal sex can be extremely painful and can even result in a physical tear or *'lesion'* in your ass. The English saying *'One in the bum, no harm done!'* is not always true.

De-armoring the Anus

Just as you would de-armour your vagina before having tantric sex, you also need to de-armour your anus in order to have pleasurable anal sex.

---

2. https://www.psychologytoday.com/us/blog/women-who-stray/201102/back-door-psychology?page=2

3. https://www.refinery29.com/en-us/does-anal-sex-feel-good

4. https://www.refinery29.com/en-us/switching-from-anal-to-vaginal-sex

5. https://www.healthline.com/health/healthy-sex/anal-sex-safety#how-to-practice-safe-sex

When someone is tense and has anxieties and fears, those stresses can be stored in the anus. Fear and bodily shame can often manifest as tightness in the anus. De-conditioning yourself and transcending sexual shame makes it easier to de-armour this region.

Refer back to Chapter 10 to refresh your memory on the mechanics of anal de-armouring. However, here is one thing to remember: The ass de-armouring is not so much about depth but *width*. Instead of getting your fingers, cock (or arm etc) in as deeply as possible, focus on getting the anus to gently dilate in width. Every morning you will find evidence that your anus can stretch pretty widely, and without pain.

Cleanliness

As many a gay *'bottoms'* will attest, fear of being dirty can be a big turn-off. Before you engage in anal sex (or anal de-armouring), be sure to douche your rectum... This means rinsing inside of your anus, as explained in greater detail in Chapter 10. Of course, you also want to wash outside your anus as well. Just make sure everything is *spic and span*.

For the penetrator, if you are using your fingers to de-armour your partner's anus, you might consider using tight latex or vinyl gloves (with a lot of lube). This makes clean-up easier, and the smoothness of the gloves reduces friction on the delicate skin inside the rectum. Both of you will likely enjoy the whole experience more if you can relax about cleanliness (and sharp fingernails) by using some nice, slippery gloves.

Oils Ain't Oils

Water-based lubricants are a ticking time-bomb for the anus... they quickly dry out and turn into a glue-like substance. In the vagina, water-based lube uses the woman's natural lubrication to sustain their slipperiness. However, as the ass has little additional source of moisture, they can quickly feel like someone left an old gummy bear up your butt to rot.

Silicon lubricant or a plant-based oil; such as coconut oil or vegetable shortening are what you are looking for. *Crisco* is legendary in gay culture for good reasons. It never dries up. You can find silicone lube and Crisco in sex shops or online.[6] Here's a good tip: grocery stores also sell Crisco (try the baking aisle), at a fraction of the cost of sex-shops. Just explain to the check-out lady if she raises an eyebrow when you take the super jumbo-sized tub, tell her you need it for a big baking contest you're planning to enter. A more truthful response may raise both eyebrows!

Start Slow, for God's Sake!

When you first enter the *'tradesman's entrance'*, proceed slowly and keep whatever you inserted (penis, dildo, finger), still for a while. You're not checking your oil level, here! Allow the ass to get used to the stretch, and don't move until it feels relaxed and pleasant. If you feel some pain in the *old chocolate starfish*, push out (like when you are on the toilet) and try not to pucker up.

You've probably seen some pretty intense porn scenes where someone starts banging away in another person's ass, but bear in mind that many porn actors have had extensive experience with anal sex. They probably have been de-armoured through years of intense ass play... or have taken some really good drugs!

When you first have anal sex, you want to start on a frustratingly-slow speed. Believe me, too slow is better than too fast. Save that fast in-and-out friction sex for later. Once you are genuinely enjoying that slow, deep anal sex, you will be able to try faster friction later.

Oh! Here's another useful tip, before I forget. If you notice her toes curling up with every pump, try taking her pantyhose off first!

Anal Orgasms

Yes, there is medical evidence that the anus can indeed feel very orgasmic through the pelvic floor nerve.

Although penile stimulation orgasms are associated with 4–8 pelvic muscle contractions, prostatic massage orgasms are associated with 12 contractions. Prostatic massage orgasms are thought to be more intense and diffuse than penile stimulation orgasms, but they require time and practice and are not liked

---

6. Please keep in mind that oils (such as coconut or Crisco) shouldn't be used with latex condoms because they can break down the latex and therefore cause the condom to break. However, silicone-based lubes are safe to use with all condoms (latex or polyurethane) and any latex product (dams, gloves, etc.)

by many men.[7] —Amjad Alwaal, M.D., M.Sc. Benjamin N. Breyer, M.D. and Tom F. Lue, M.D.b

Ass Communication

While anal sex is quite high on most people's fantasies, many people are afraid to *'pop their partner*'s pooper' because they are afraid to hurt them. If your partner wishes to have anal sex, you can ask them to verbally encourage you. Not only will this help you overcome the stigma that you are doing something wrong, but it will give you confirmation that your partner is *enthusiastically* consenting... which is always a good thing.[8] The clearer they are with their words, the easier this will be for you to know how it's really going.

Does it hurt?

A little... but it feels good, too. Can you just keep it in there and let me relax for a little bit?

Yes. I can do that. How does it feel now?

Good, yes. Now a little bit more... but slooooowly.

Sure. Is this slow enough?

Yes. Now can you go a little bit faster?

Etc., etc.

Seeing your partner enjoying themselves and hearing them asking you enthusiastically to pump their ass harder can be quite a pleasant interaction, for all concerned. The more they talk and the more they encourage you, the less you will have to guess what they need. Empathy is important, but communication also builds trust. Over time, you may be able to use more non-verbal cues such as moans, groans (and screams), instead of words.

Have Fun, and Don't Take it Too Seriously.

I've given you some guidelines here. However, if this is new for you, you might be tempted to use this chapter as a technical manual. Poke here, hold there, stretch, communicate... got it! But remember, *this is supposed*

7. https://www.ncbi.nlm.nih.gov/pmc/articles/PMC4896089/

8. https://www.salon.com/2014/08/14/young_men_dont_think_they_need_consent_for_anal_sex/

to be fun. Don't start this whole process with the expectation of achieving porn-style butt sex on the first go. Just like the first time you pick up a banjo, don't expect to be able to play the *Deliverance*, duelling-banjos tune. All forms of tantric sex are best when they are goal-free. Yes, the anus can have a long, valley-like orgasm through the pelvic floor nerve for all genders, but actively seeking this tantric orgasm will, in most cases, overload the user and turn the excess horniness into a pudendal nerve orgasm.

Anal Sex as a Path to Enlightenment?

OK, so you're probably not going to achieve Nirvana just because you've had a dick in your butt... but one thing is for certain, being the recipient of anal sex teaches you how to be in the receptive, submissive position. There is no better way to develop empathy than by having the same shared experience. Just as great dominatrixes often start out in the submissive role, if you want to be great at anal sex, a good place to start is by learning how to join the *doughnut defecation program* yourself.

Photo credit: *Bpcraddock* (https://pixabay.com/users/bpcraddock-305024/), https://pixabay.com/photos/sign-street-road-road-signs-2454791/

32

I KNOW HOW TO TOUCH

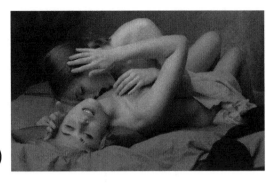

Analysing Good Touch

With the right touch, women can experience more subtle orgasms through the bodily senses via the Vagus nerve in ways that men cannot.[1,2]

Good Touch/Bad Touch

Have you ever had someone grab your nipple out of nowhere and just start twirling it around like someone trying to tune in an old-style radio? Or stick their tongue in your ear and gift you with a 'wet-willy' before you were aroused? Maybe you had someone start rubbing on your clit before you were horny and it felt more like nails on a chalkboard than bagels on Sunday. If you are a woman, chances are you answered 'yes' to all of the above. If you're a man, have you had someone grab your penis with a death grip and start jackhammering without forewarning? I know these are rather extreme examples of bad touch, but my point is that getting touched right is pretty damn important, maybe only second to good hygiene. You can easily figure out how to have good hygiene, but how do you learn to touch better? To answer that, let's start with two of the biggest complaints: Too fast and too greedy.

---

1. https://www.wired.com/2007/01/exploring-the-mind-body-orgasm/

2. https://www.huffpost.com/entry/what-do-singing-throats-a_b_268642

Greedy Touch

Greedy touch can be gross, and most of the perpetrators who do it don't realise that's how it's being received. It seems that, as soon as there is an end goal, the destination becomes more important than the journey. The sexual conveyor belt starts, and you are processed like a Ford Model T. Let's start with some kissing, touch a boob over the shirt, touch a boob under the shirt, a finger here, a tongue there... Check, check, check! Now she's wet enough for the grand entrance of the penis.[3]

Having spent time in both male and female modes, and having interacted sexually with both genders, I can say there is a quite dramatic difference in just how much touch can vary. As a generalisation, lesbian sex is usually a bit more sensitive and free-flowing than heterosexual sex. Lesbian sex tends to include more energetic sex and is often less focused on genitals. Sex with men can have an interesting quality of greediness, which can be quite horny in itself when you feel someone is really into you. However, non-mutual greediness can feel akin to being molested.

Slow Your Roll, Bruh!

Regardless of you being a man or a woman, if you are unsure how to touch your partner in a way that brings them pleasure, here's a winning formula. Slow down your touch by 20%. Most people move too quickly. Over time, we have all learned to move at the most efficient pace possible. If you live in a city, you probably walk quickly, talk quickly and you might even eat quickly. However, we obviously don't want to touch our partner as if we were commuting to work or gobbling down a ham sandwich on our 30-minute lunch break. Touch like you are on vacation and you want this moment to last forever. Remember, the Caribbean *'go slow bro'* mantra will allow you time to smell the flowers (or whatever odours waft your way).[4]

Same Old, Same Old

It's easy to get into a routine, even for those who are quite skilled at sex. The reason is that if we did something that worked last time, there's a

---

3. https://www.mic.com/articles/110374/
   the-four-bases-system-is-everything-wrong-with-how-we-talk-about-sex

4. https://www.psychologytoday.com/us/blog/shameless-woman/201009/
   what-is-organic-orgasm

big temptation to try and repeat that star performance for more beloved brownie points. We all know it's possible to get lazy and stuck in a rut, especially when we've been with the same partner for a while. A repetitive roadmap technique becomes quickly predictable, and thus boring.[5]

You want to flow with whatever their body evokes from you. Try not to think about what you're doing or what you are going to do next, but rather the active meditation of witnessing your hands move. Pay attention to the kind of response your touch elicits and ask each other not to fake anything. In this way, you'll keep the feedback authentic and your compass will continue pointing towards true North. If your partner seems more like a sack of potatoes than popping popcorn, you might want to switch it up little.

The best kind of sex is like a double-blind experiment where both parties don't actually know what touch is going to happen in the next moment. It's like a horizontal ecstatic dance.[6] The person doing the touching seems to be in control, but they are really taking the cues from the responses of the one being touched.[7]

Touch Talk

Everyone is different, so the easiest way to learn how to touch a new lover is to ask while you are touching them. The type of touch that someone wants, can change from one moment to the next. Initially, they may want a firm-but-gentle touch. Then, they may want a very light touch in some specific areas, for example, on the inside of the arm, or on the side of the neck. As things get hot and heavy, a bit more playful and rough can also work. Variety is a great interest-sustainer.

Stay present to perceive all the cues: visual, verbal and physical. The receiver's job is to make sure their non-verbal responses are obvious enough for the other to be able to navigate. Women seem to be better at reading more subtle clues than men, and often mistakenly expect the same level of perception. If he touches you in a way that you like, then give a non-verbal clue like a moan to encourage him to go more in that direction. Think of it as a game of hot and cold. If his touch leaves you cold, then mimic a dead

5. https://www.cosmopolitan.com/sex-love/advice/a1846/bust-out-of-a-sex-rut/

6. https://www.wellandgood.com/what-is-ecstatic-dance/

7. https://www.livescience.com/14498-emerging-adults-empathy-sexual-health-satisfaction.html

I KNOW HOW TO TOUCH

fish and see if that gives him a prod towards a better direction. It may start off a little mechanical, but once you get into the swing of things, it will turn into a fluid back-and-forth exchange of information through touch. Instead of having three or four moves, now you have many possible ways of touching, of being touched and of reacting to touch. In this way, sex can be vastly different every time you engage. No more boring, repetitive sex moves. Instead, sex can become more fresh and interesting.

Finally, don't be stingy with your responses if you are being touched well. The response is the *reward* for all the work being done by the initiator.

33

I KNOW HOW TO HAVE SEX

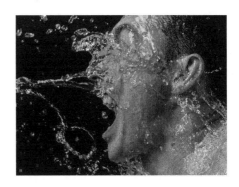

Doubt is the Seed of Learning

Here's a common snippet of a casual conversation with someone I've just met:

So, what do you do for work?

I'm writing an educational book about sex.

Oh for teenagers...

No for adults like yourself.

Oh... I think I know how to have sex... it's pretty idiot-proof, right?

At which point I resist the temptation to prove them an idiot. From past experience, that usually doesn't end well. I am more likely to end up like the guy in the photo above... with his G&T in my face.

One of the painful things about our time is that those who feel certainty are stupid, and those with any imagination and understanding are filled with doubt and indecision. —Bertrand Russell (1872-1970), English philosopher

Many people routinely watching the world of *'friction-only sex'* porn are constantly being reassured that this is the totality of sexual possibilities. I have no moral judgement against porn, it's just that it is not the best tantric sex teacher. Using porn as a sex manual is like trying to learn how to drive a car by watching *The Fast and the Furious!*

There are a few problems related to watching porn regularly,[1,2] but the main reason I don't advocate the regular use of porn is that it tends to hyper-stimulate the visual cortex. Over-stimulating the brain with a large variety of rapidly-changing images has been shown to de-sensitise us as lovers in real life. Instead of being fully present with our lovers, we can become less able to feel sexually stimulated by our normal, slower reality and therefore need to rely on fantasies in our head. Repetitive porn-viewing can create a safe *'keyhole observer'* witness: A safe position that doesn't require you to be in the picture. So, when we finally get IRL with another flesh-puppet, we may need to keep activating our visual cortex with internal fantasies. The risk is that if you do so, you are then forced to disconnect from your lover in order to get hot (or hard).[3,4] The result is that we become less capable of being present as we close our eyes to the real world.

If you want to practise greater control and still choose to watch porn, I would recommend at least stopping before the *'money shot'*. Just seeing the image of a penis ejaculating can act like a little sex virus in the mind, stimulating that addiction and making it difficult to control yourself—even hours later. It's like being on a diet and then watching your co-workers eat birthday cake... or hanging around drinkers and smokers if you have recently quit.

Porn and Love

There is some early (but inconclusive) research on how the brain reacts to excessive viewing of pornography. In summary, this research advocates that watching porn seems to rewire your brain in such a way that you become more obsessive, less sensitive, less empathetic and less capable of noticing beauty and experiencing love.

Just as drug addicts need increasingly higher doses of drugs, people

1. https://www.psychologytoday.com/us/blog/all-about-sex/201208/
    the-real-problem-porn-its-bad-sex

2. https://aifs.gov.au/sites/default/files/publication-documents/rr_the_effects_of_
    pornography_on_children_and_young_people_1.pdf

3. https://www.psychologytoday.com/us/blog/love-and-sex-in-the-digital-age/201401/
    is-male-porn-use-ruining-sex

4. Kühn S, Gallinat J. *Brain Structure and Functional Connectivity Associated With Pornography Consumption: The Brain on Porn.* JAMA Psychiatry. 2014;71(7):827–834. doi:https://doi.
    org/10.1001/jamapsychiatry.2014.93

with a regular porn watching habit seem to need increasingly higher levels of visual sexual stimulation (and novelty) in order to reach the same level of arousal. Over time, this hunger for stimulation craves more unusual and extreme videos.

There are many contradicting opinions from researchers on the claims above and on whether or not there is such a thing called *porn addiction*. I'm not judging anyone here and I don't want to argue this point as I simply don't know. I can only speak from my own empirical knowledge as well as what I've heard from thousands of TNT workshop participants who shared their experiences with me.

If you want to know more about this subject I suggest you conduct your own internet research and make up your own mind.

Tantra Porn?

You know what doesn't look exciting and horny? Watching no-friction sex. Very few want to jack off to two people opening their hearts up to each other and connecting deeply. The problem is that the lack of kinaesthetic feeling capacity of a camera means it's incapable of recording internal tantric subtleties. It's the things that you *can't* see that are the most interesting when you're having tantric sex. The exchange of energy, how it circulates inside the body, how it feels to have your cervix pressed kindly, etc. So for me, it is the same as watching sport on TV; I'd rather be playing it myself.

As a side note, The New Tantra has created educational tantric porn in the form of step-by-step guided videos of basic and advanced tantric sexual skills. The intention of these explicit videos is for people to learn how to improve their physical sensitivity and explore deeper forms of tantric sex at home, not orientated towards ejaculation or entertainment.[5]

Sex is Messy

Porn is also not good for realistic expectations on the ease of safe sex. It never shows the reality of how to put on condoms or how to figure out the right moment to grab one. In porn, it seems that condoms just appear magically on the penis. Ever seen one being rolled-on in your private late-night viewing, or the messy clean up that comes afterwards?

---

5. https://courses.thenewtantra.com

It gets even worse when there are multiple partners in the same scene. It's not horny to watch people changing out condoms before swapping holes. It's not sexy to see people washing their hands between partners, sanitising their hands with Alcogel or cleaning toys with Barbicide. These essential (but unsexy) aspects of safe and healthy sex play are (understandably) omitted.

Another major omission in porn is the impact of peak orgasm on the way we feel. The slumping into a lifeless heap a few minutes after the man ejaculates or the subtle feeling of shame after the regular orgasm. The sudden feeling of *loss of interest in the other* are not exactly high-rated money makers! Have you ever noticed how quickly the scene is cut after ejaculation? *'Money shot'* porn doesn't exactly offer you a window into an alternative way of practising sex that leaves you feeling happy, horny and creative. This is no judgemental, moral finger-wagging from my side... I'm just pointing out some tantric affects to consider.

Photo credit: *David Pinocy* (https://www.shutterstock.com/g/davidpinocy),
https://www.shutterstock.com/image-photo/big-splash-man-face-789796696

34
ROMANCE IS GOOD

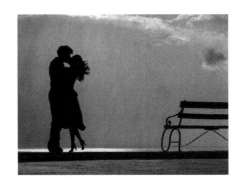

Feminine Porn...
The Romantic Dream

This book has no intentions of being a book about relationship coaching, per se. As the title states, it's about sex. As one of my deepest long-term teachers—Mykonos—once said to me *Never advise on relationships; it's a can of worms*. Wise advice, indeed! I certainly don't feel qualified to teach in that field. It's not within the scope of this book to give advice on how to make relationships work. There are other books for that. Perhaps, the only tie-in between the two is that having a strong tantric sexual base creates the sexual bonding and physical foundation that allows us to do the necessary emotional relationship work.

There are some good relationship coaches out there, but having met a lot of teachers in our fields, I rarely meet one that has mastered both. Yes, there are some who have managed to become really good, caring, loving friends and have good tools to recommend to others. Most of them seemed to have a good regular sex life at the start, but managing to sustain both a good sex life and a good relationship in the long-term (especially with kids), is exceptionally rare, unless you combine relationship skills with tantra.

The reason I say this is not to be cynical, but if people make false claims that a good relationship bond *automatically* equates to great sex, they are perhaps unintentionally supporting a romantic myth that one produces the other. The reason I even mention the romantic dream in a book about sex is because it can certainly limit the ability to practise tantric sex. Let me explain: in a heterosexual scenario, sexual shame and *waiting for romantic love from Mr Right* limits women's sexual exploration, and coincidentally, dries up the supply of tantric females for straight men.

Honey Trap

The romantic dream is probably the single riskiest area for feminine delusion. Remember, I am using the term *'feminine'* in a non-gender way throughout this book... any person with a predominantly feminine nature can fall into this trap.

Many of us have either been there or witnessed a friend going through the romantic delusion. It's easy to get stuck in a cycle of hoping to be saved by the *knight in shining armour* rather than working through problems, or blaming others when our lives don't work out the way we want.[1] Rather than figuring out what lies at the root of our unhappiness and addressing the issue, we might mistakenly believe that bringing the perfect person into our lives will *cure* our problems. It seems it's less demanding to unconsciously outsource our emotional state to others than to actually rectify our own problems. This creates *victim mentality* and renders us powerless to change the situation because we have just removed ourselves from the equation.

The Rapunzel Complex

Obviously, there's nothing wrong with healthy romance and finding creative ways to demonstrate our love to our partner. The romantic dream I am talking about is when a person believes that their life would be perfect *'only if'* a new lover would come along and sweep them off their feet and save them.[2]

The familiar story of Rapunzel can alternatively be seen as a woman trapped by her blindness to see her capabilities and resources. Surely, if she could let her hair down for someone else to save her, she could have cut her own hair off and used it as a rope to climb down the tower herself. (Didn't think of that one when you were 7 years old, did you?)

The romantic dream comes in many forms and with various underlying

---

1. https://www.yourtango.com/experts/
   david-wygant/4-reasons-man-your-dreams-doesn-t-exist

2. https://everydayfeminism.com/2014/10/savior-complex-toxic-relationship/

motives. Some people search for someone to provide them with security so they can stop working, stay at home and have babies.[3] Other people want a rich partner so they can travel the world, or a younger lover to make them feel young again. There is nothing wrong with any of those scenarios, *per se*. The main issue arises when we put our lives on hold, waiting for someone else to fix us. Placing our happiness in someone else's hands usually ends in demanding the other to fulfil us and, conversely, feeling *anger* if they don't deliver. There is nothing more unattractive than *neediness*[4] or its more aggressive cousin, *entitlement*.[5]

Unrealistic expectations can set up the all-too-common dynamics of complaining.[6] As soon as the other is unable to meet our needs, we feel we have the right to demand them to change. It seems we must all cut off our own ponytails and climb out of prison ourselves.

We are probably familiar with the feeling of when love goes bad. One person is unhappy, and they believe that their partner must suffer alongside them. Sometimes, you see people who were recently claiming to deeply love and care for each other, now ensuing in bitter arguments in divorce court. It makes one doubt the sincerity of newly proclaimed love.

Photo credit: *Dimitris Vetsikas* (https://pixabay.com/users/dimitrisvetsikas1969-1857980/), https://pixabay.com/photos/couple-romance-love-kiss-lovers-3064048/

3. https://www.stuff.co.nz/life-style/love-sex/72632931/
    men-want-beauty-women-want-financial-security-from-relationships

4. https://www.psychologytoday.com/us/blog/the-intelligent-divorce/201208/
    who-wants-be-needy-six-solutions

5. https://www.aconsciousrethink.com/4561/5-ways-sense-entitlement-reveals/

6. https://www.psychologytoday.com/us/blog/meet-catch-and-keep/201705/
    expectations-can-hurt-your-relationship

35

CALLING A WOMAN A 'SLUT' IS DEROGATORY

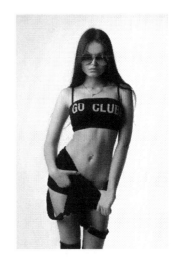

Well, Yes, it Can Be, But...

Allow me, if you will, to propose the argument that one can call a woman a slut (with her consent) as a compliment. Of course, you should never call a woman by any name that she perceives as demeaning, negatively objectifying, or insulting. *SlutWalk* has correctly stood up against people using this word in a derogatory way.[1,2] My point is that there is an alternative use of the word *'slut'* that can be applicable in tantric practice to liberate a woman's wilder aspects.

A slut is a woman who really enjoys sex, so much so that she ignores the rules of society with unabashed enjoyment of sex. In Western countries, the self-identified slut is progressively becoming an icon representing the power that women take back when they revel in their own sexuality and pleasure.[3] When you use this word in bed, the negative connotations and the taboo associated with it can be highly erotic *for the woman*, when both parties know it is being done with respect.

1. https://msmagazine.com/2015/10/09/amber-roses-feminism-for-women-who-have-been-through-shit/

2. https://time.com/4961144/amber-rose-slut-walk-essay/

3. https://www.vogue.com.au/culture/features/karley-sciortino-of-slutever-on-reclaiming-the-word-slut/news-story/8da2ff561c5c2301345821b411e3b6a7

Playing in the dark verbal spectrum of *labels* can help her access the raw sexual energy that can be locked in the most extreme forms of feminine archetypes. Most women have been conditioned to repress their sexuality. The actions of concerned parents, training girls to avoid dressing or behaving in a sexually enticing way, can have a lifelong effect. *'Don't wear that skirt, darling. It's way too short.'* Of course, all of this was based on good intentions, as sadly there *can* be physical and social repercussions for young women who are openly sexual, but oftentimes those protective comments unconsciously limit the sexual potential of an otherwise free-thinking, adult woman.[4]

Conditioning comes not only from parents, religion and society but perhaps even more powerfully from peers.[5] Girls can be as cruel emotional bullies as boys can be physical ones. Of course, we never hear the sexual-promiscuity insult used between boys.[6] Boys who bed a lot of girls are *'studs'* and considered cool. It is kind of unfair (and probably one reason why transsexuals don't have the same slut-shaming conditioning as women often have).

Disempowering Women Unintentionally

The brilliant feminist Camille Paglia points out that whilst the #metoo movement has led to many positive and needed reforms, it can also produce the undesired effect of disempowering women.[7] By making white, upper-class women feel they need institutions to protect them, it can send the unspoken message that they don't have the power to say *'no!'* in the moment.

If women expect equal treatment in society, they must stop asking for infantilising special protections. With freedom comes personal responsibility. —Camille Paglia.[8]

Similarly, the shadow side of the feminist movement is the loss of some of

---

4. https://www.huffpost.com/entry/the-truth-about-slut-shaming_b_7054162

5. https://www.theatlantic.com/health/archive/2014/05/theres-no-such-thing-as-a-slut/371773/

6. https://www.ncbi.nlm.nih.gov/pmc/articles/PMC4256532/

7. https://womenintheworld.com/2018/02/27/camille-paglia-slams-counterproductive-metoo-movement-warns-women-to-speak-up-now-or-shut-up-later/

8. https://www.eurozine.com/the-feminist-moment/

the positive aspects of gender difference and labels. If we are to reclaim the healthy aspects of the word *'slut'*, we need to de-condition some of our hidden assumptions. We have the opportunity to support women to openly admit that they enjoy sex, without suffering any negative connotations. Women don't need to be chaste to be deserving of respect, and the opposite is also true. You don't have to treat a woman like she is *pure as the driven snow'* to respect her. In fact, being able to use edgy labels in a positive way can support your female partner to claim her full, sexual, feminine spectrum. That's why back in 2010 I added the word *'divine'* to *'slut'* to help differentiate two uses of the same word, to clarify the positive aspects and less shaming of liberal women.

When Does Sex Get Too Nice?

Unfortunately, the lighter shade of the spectrum is usually the limit of the mainstream's understanding of tantra. On many occasions, I've heard people saying *'Yes, we did tantra for a while, but he got bored after a few months'*. Of course! Cuddling and connecting in the heart are important aspects of a healthy sex life, but limiting sex to the flavours of *mother* or *virgin* is comparable to limiting the woman to wearing only one set of earrings for a year.

Conversely, if men get scared of stronger feminine flavours and are unable to respond to a wide variety of feminine energy, their partners may understandably get bored. In the same fashion, men often get bored and look elsewhere if their feminine lovers only provide one or two flavours of the large spectrum of feminine potential.

Sacred Slut

In Chapter 12, we discussed polarity. We talked about how the average man has a lot more to learn when it comes to flowing between the masculine and feminine modes in an average day. This is because most women are used to embodying masculine and feminine qualities in order to navigate the world, while men can often get away with using mainly their masculine qualities. While women may have experience with both polarities in their daily lives, they may need further development in the area of moving between polarities in bed and in intimate relationships. The energy of the sacred slut is a very specific flavour that usually requires a deeper layer of freedom beyond what is openly accepted by a parochial society.

Not everyone is capable of letting-go easily. It can be difficult to get into a state of relaxation and horniness when some part of our minds are overly concerned with something nagging, like an overdue phone bill. This is where teamwork and support from someone else can help direct us into a state of surrender and vulnerability. Reclaiming the word *slut* can help support the much needed liberation of the wild and passionate end of the feminine spectrum.

Photo credit: *Khusen Rustamov* (https://pixabay.com/users/xusenru-1829710/), https://pixabay.com/photos/girl-in-overalls-jumpsuit-shorts-1741733/

36

SPIRITUAL PEOPLE ARE NONSEXUAL

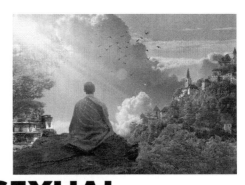

Guru Myths

Every Easter in San Francisco, there is an event called the Hunky Jesus Contest,[1] hosted by a group called the Sisters of Perpetual Indulgence.[2] Participants dress as various types of Jesuses such as *'Wet T-Shirt Jesus'*, *'Stripper Jesus'* and *'Sweet Jesus'*—whose costume is candy-themed.[3] This event attracts a lot of attention and, obviously, a substantial amount of criticism, to the point of being labelled as *'sacrilegious'*. Let's take a closer look at why this event is considered so blasphemous. Besides the indignity of portraying the Son of God as someone who shakes their booty for cash, the mere thought that Jesus may not have been celibate seems inconceivable for most people. Thinking of holy people having sex is such a taboo that sexualising Jesus is completely out of bounds for believers.

Suppressing Sexual Desire Doesn't Work

The myriad of holy-looking spiritual men in history makes it easy to build the picture that enlightenment is exclusively non-sexual. In the Christian tradition, not only is there Jesus but also Joseph and Mary and the immaculate conception. Any suggestions that Jesus may have had brothers or

---

1. https://sfist.com/2019/04/22/hunky-jesus-contest-returns-to-dolores-park-for-sisters-of-perpetual-indulgences-40th-anniversary/

2. History of The Sisters of Perpetual Indulgence. https://www.thesisters.org/sistory

3. https://sfist.com/2017/04/17/hunky_jesus_title_goes_to_wet_t-shi/

sisters is considered heresy.[4]

As an article in *The Economist* rightly points out, it would be one thing if religious leaders were selected from people who have chosen celibacy because they have already transcended sexual urges. However, as they are expected to take on celibacy as an act of self-sacrifice or simply as a form of repression, it seems inevitable for problems to arise.[5]

Perhaps this approach of using self-discipline to control sexual urges forces some spiritual leaders to create a false persona that they are un-interested in sex. The plethora of sex-abuse cases in the Catholic Church is highly likely to be a symptom of the problems created by suppression.[6] Priests and nuns are required to hide their sexual desires and, at the same time, they are entrusted with unsupervised access to the most vulnerable people in the community, women and children.[7,8]

But let's not jump on the new-age bandwagon and bash religion. There is a lot of good intentions behind many of the issues, and on the whole it seems that religion does its best. The original aim of religion is probably not to suppress sexuality. Sexuality regulation is a means to an end. The real aim of religion is to avoid violence and competition getting out of hand and spiral into all out war. And since women have traditionally been the main reason for male aggressive competition, in both animals and humans, religion may well be attempting to regulate that urge.

This concept that *'virtuous people do not desire sex'* is pervasive in our society. In my opinion, virtually all forms of spirituality in our culture are nothing more than intentions to be spiritual through changing the thinking processes, without any deeper transformation happening. The result of this *'mind over flesh'* approach can easily lead to suppression and self-shaming. What I consider being spiritual is the *transcendence of mind*, which is some-thing entirely different.

4.   https://www.catholic.com/magazine/online-edition/jesus-had-brothers

5.   *The Economist* explains, Why Catholic priests practise celibacy https://www.economist.com/the-economist-explains/2017/03/23/why-catholic-priests-practise-celibacy

6.   https://www.bbc.com/news/topics/c9z6w6n469et/catholic-church-sexual-abuse-cases

7.   https://www.npr.org/2019/05/30/722119046/survivors-of-sexual-abuse-by-nuns-want-greater-visibility-for-their-claims

8.   https://www.pbs.org/newshour/show/abused-nuns-reveal-stories-of-rape-forced-abortions

There is more wisdom in your body than in your deepest philosophy. —Friedrich Nietzsche, Thus Spoke Zarathustra

Satori

The Encyclopaedia Britannica defines Satori as *'The inner, intuitive experience of Enlightenment... indescribable, and unintelligible by reason and logic.'*[9] In my experience, satori is something akin to a temporary enlightenment... a taste of being one with everything in which the usual feeling of being separate from our surroundings becomes momentarily suspended... and tantra sex seems to be the the strongest way to experience that transcendence naturally.

...transcendent sex, in the way I define it, is when sex or sexual activity triggers an altered state; and by that I mean some sense of change in your sense of self. Your sense of self may expand. It could be out of your normal body which most of us think of as a part of ourselves. It could be larger than yourself. It could be that you feel interconnected with all beings. It could be a sense of change in time or space. —Jenny Wade, developmental psychologist, author of *'Transcendent sex.'*[10]

The feeling of *'myself'* as a limited and separate consciousness is then experienced as never actually being separate from the world of Consciousness itself. In other words, an experience in which consciousness recognises its own indivisibility, like being in a dream in which there is no doer and no separate observer behind the eyes.

I'm not saying that reality is an illusion or that there is a deeper reality or claim for any kind of nirvana heavenly state, I am saying that the world we see *is* heavenly if we didn't feel so disconnected and inherently separate from it every waking moment. That's what I like about Tantra, it is down-to-earth and gives awesome tools to deal with all the mundane stuff we need to deal with in daily life, as well as expand our limited sense of self and give us greater capacity to function day-to-day.

When we are freed from *self-reflection* the body can enter a *flow state* that I call *non-interference*. The body acts without habituated or planned actions about what to do next. A kind of light-hearted playful surrender.

---

9. https://www.britannica.com/topic/Satori
10. https://www.psychologytoday.com/us/blog/the-empowerment-diary/201609/ what-you-should-know-about-transcending-during-sex

Lovemaking is one of the strongest expressions of opposites in union—the One expressing Itself through the archetypal Masculine and Feminine in human form.

In that mindless playing-field, sex can acquire an almost magic-like quality, as if it comes from a deeper source of intelligence than the regular mind. The new and innocent, mindless sexual expression moves away from the impulses of greed, relief and incessant pleasure-seeking toward a *'why not celebrate?'* and *'how can I share this state with someone else through physical intimacy?'*

I hope this kind of pure sexuality is not unbecoming of a spiritually-attained person, especially if they are doing it as a gift to another? If it were, the most highly evolved people on this planet would not spread their talents and genes to their offspring... which seems a like a bit of a waste!

Photo credit: *Inactive user 4144132* (https://pixabay.com/users/4144132-4144132/), https://pixabay.com/photos/meditation-buddhism-monk-temple-2214532/

37

WE SHOULD ONLY HAVE SEX WITH LOVE

It's Complicated...

Sex with love seems to be the best combination for most people. I think few would argue that there are many things in life better than great sex with someone you love. However, what can we do when we are not in the rare position of having sex with someone we are in love with? Should we abstain?

Let's be realistic, we don't find someone to fall in love with every day. Perhaps it's even virtually impossible for people to love a partner truly before they have spent a lot of time and effort on their own development. Finding two people that love each other unconditionally as we do our children, seems exceedingly rare these days.[1]

Sex with Love is Ideal

In general, committed, long-term relationships provide the best environment for tantric sex. Not having to search for new love partners is safer, less time-consuming, and makes for a deeper experience. However, if you don't have anyone special, doesn't it still make sense to be available for tantric sexual practice and sexual yoga with someone even if you're not in love with them? Practising tantric sex with good, caring people and clear

---

1. https://psychcentral.com/blog/a-parents-unconditional-love/

intentions can prepare us for the experience of tantric sex within a relationship. It's probably a more productive preparation than celibacy.

While having sex with someone you love would be ideal, tantric practice dates can help us shed the shame of being sexual creatures hidden behind a mask of social propriety. It allows both sexes more opportunities to practice transcending sex fixations.[2]

Regular Sex is a Trap

Regular sex is not a good vehicle if you want to grow, develop and transcend superficial fantasies. Think of all the effort it might take to find the right people to fulfil that specific scenario you longed for. It takes a lot of work (and luck) to fully live out a fantasy. As I mentioned before, the trick is to find caring, responsible and loving people to help you create the fantasy scenario and hold on to the horniest sustainable moment until you feel satiated, which usually occurs just before the spasm-orgasm sets off the pumping contractions. If the spasm reflex hits before you are satiated, you will lose that delicious maximum horny energy. Spending as much time at maximum horniness right before the orgasm is the key.[3]

While having sex without the requirement for love can be a part of a relaxed tantric education, *'Too much of a good thing is good for nothing!'* Men can be more susceptible to getting stuck in the endless exploration of loveless sex, as masculine people generally find it easier to separate sex from their feelings. In general, women often have the opposite tendency, usually experiencing feelings and sex far more entwined. For this reason, enjoying sex without shame and breaking the socially-acceptable *'good girl'* requirement of only having sex with someone who matches their romantic dream, can be a liberating experience.[4,5,6]

The good news is that agendas merge with practice. Tantrically mature

2. https://www.psychologytoday.com/us/blog/women-who-stray/201708/overcoming-religious-sexual-shame

3. https://www.health.com/sex/edging-sex

4. https://positivepsychology.com/shame-resilience-theory/

5. https://www.psychologytoday.com/us/blog/compassion-matters/201306/misconceptions-about-womans-sexuality

6. Clark, Noel. 'The etiology and phenomenology of sexual shame: A grounded theory study.' (2017). http://digitalcommons.spu.edu/cgi/viewcontent.cgi?article=1024&context=cpy_etd

men who know they are sexually competent and have lived out their sexual urges generally move toward more connected and loving sex as *quantity* is replaced by *quality*. Problem solved.

Photo credit: *Stokpic* (https://pixabay.com/users/stokpic-692575/), https://pixabay.com/photos/couple-making-out-young-people-731890/

38

APHRODISIACS ARE A MYTH

Sexual
Stimulants

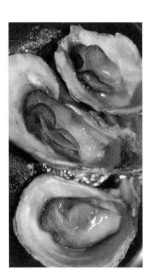

In my exploratory days, I tried countless commercial aphrodisiacs that failed to live up to their advertised promises. In fact, the only noticeable effect was on my wallet. There is little clinical merit to the claims that sex-shop aphrodisiacs actually work.[1] Unfortunately, the opposite is blatantly true, as there are many factors known to *decrease* libido.[2]

If you don't feel as horny as you would like, rest assured that you are not alone. Loss of libido seems to be a problem for many people.[3] Men often experience decreased libido over time due to lower levels of testosterone. This can also be commonly associated with a general lack of drive and passion for life, and even depression.[4] One remedy is to increase testosterone. This can be done naturally through regular exercise, losing weight, getting sufficient sleep and consuming Vitamin D, Zinc and moderating caffeine intake.[5] If none of these work, testosterone replacement therapy is quicker solution, but be aware of negative side effects to this more direct

1. https://www.mayoclinic.org/healthy-lifestyle/sexual-health/expert-answers/natural-aphrodisiacs/faq-20058252

2. https://www.nhs.uk/conditions/loss-of-libido/

3. https://www.nhsinform.scot/illnesses-and-conditions/sexual-and-reproductive/loss-of-libido

4. https://www.webmd.com/men/how-low-testosterone-can-affect-your-sex-drive#1

5. https://www.healthline.com/health/low-testosterone/testosterone-replacement-therapy-and-other-options#takeaway

approach.[6] Testosterone injections can halt its natural production in the testes and even cause the *'old boys'* to shrink over time. A more sustainable solution is taking supplements that provide enough nutrients for the body to produce this hormone naturally.

Stress, anxiety, depression and chronic lack of sleep can also reduce the level of passion for both genders.[7] This is an unfortunate catch-22, as sex is a fun exercise and known to be a great natural way to reduce many of these negative issues.[8,9] Antidepressants such as selective serotonin reuptake inhibitors, fluoxetine (Prozac), paroxetine (Paxil), fluvoxamine (Luvox), citalopram (Celexa) and sertraline (Zoloft) are known to reduce sex drive.[10,11,12]

Although there doesn't seem to be any effective commercial aphrodisiacs, there are illegal drugs that make you want to rip your lover's clothes off and do the *'horizontal boogie'* all night long.[13] Drugs such as GHB, amphetamines and cocaine are often used as sexual stimulants, despite their many downsides, including an increased risk of exposure to HIV due to reckless behaviour.[14]

My take on this is that most illegal aphrodisiacs are illegal for a good reason. The side-effects to their users and the people around them make them a bad long-term choice. While some substances can appear to act as a temporary spiritual accelerator, in the long-run, natural is best. I'm certainly not against the occasional use of people having an outlet in a legal, conscious and careful manner. Every society needs a relaxant—such

6. https://www.health.harvard.edu/mens-health/is-testosterone-therapy-safe-take-a-breath-before-you-take-the-plunge

7. https://www.psychologytoday.com/us/blog/the-truth-about-exercise-addiction/201808/the-connection-between-sex-and-sleep

8. https://www.verywellmind.com/sex-as-a-stress-management-technique-3144601

9. Lastella M, O'Mullan C, Paterson JL, Reynolds AC. Sex and Sleep: Perceptions of Sex as a Sleep Promoting Behavior in the General Adult Population. *Front Public Health*. 2019;7:33. Published 2019 Mar 4. doi:10.3389/fpubh.2019.00033

10. https://www.aafp.org/afp/2000/0815/p782.html

11. https://www.ncbi.nlm.nih.gov/pmc/articles/PMC4816679/

12. https://www.psychologytoday.com/us/blog/all-about-sex/201902/the-latest-birth-control-pills-and-women-s-libido

13. https://www.ncbi.nlm.nih.gov/pmc/articles/PMC5771052/

14. https://www.lambeth.gov.uk/sites/default/files/ssh-chemsex-study-final-main-report.pdf

as alcohol in the West. Shamanic rituals have long been used by native indigenous cultures to transcend the normal contracted mind temporarily, and to receive a bodily imprint of greater openness. This bodily memory can then act as a type of spiritual roadmap, and be practised later on without the need of a crutch (the catalyst substance). However, for those shamanic substances I have researched, there seems to be no long-term, sustainable benefit to repeated, regular use.

The other challenge to using aphrodisiacs is that anything that artificially improves your mood will artificially depress your mood afterwards, and often for a longer time. If you have ever met someone trying to get off anti-depressants, you may understand why they are often regarded as a one-way street. This is not unlike using large amounts of alcohol to forget problems. Not a very sustainable solution. The large quantity you need to drink makes the associated hangover and long-term side-effects too high a price to pay for my liking.

A general rule of thumb is that the more unnatural and chemical derived the substance is, the higher the risk of short and long-term side-effects. A good example is ecstasy/MDMA/amphetamines. These substances might produce 10 hours of feeling *'on top of the world,'* happy, horny and connected to others, but later comes *'razor-blade Tuesday'* where people experience the exact opposite. The result is that they end up paying for that fun night with some later abject misery in which many experience depression, anxiety, aggressiveness and irritability.[15] There are also numerous scientific studies showing that these type of drugs can cause long-term damage to serotonin receptors. In other words, too many party nights with the wrong chems might make you feel permanently flatter.[16] No thanks!

There is scientific evidence that people have more sex and enjoy it more when they use marijuana.[17]

Marijuana use is very common. But its large-scale use and association with sexual frequency hasn't been studied much in a scientific way. What we found was compared to never-users, those who reported daily use had about 20 percent more sex. —Michael Eisenberg, Assistant Professor of Urology, Stanford

---

15. https://www.drugabuse.gov/publications/research-reports/mdma-ecstasy-abuse/what-are-effects-mdma

16. https://www.ncbi.nlm.nih.gov/pmc/articles/PMC1071023/

17. https://www.forbes.com/sites/sarabrittanysomerset/2018/09/10/new-studies-show-that-marijuana-enhances-and-increases-sex/#36e4fa0429d2

University

The worldwide trend to decriminalise pot gives people an alternative to alcohol (and its well-known side effects to drinkers and society). However, legalisation can also give the impression that legal = benign. Just like in the case of alcohol, legal drugs still carry risks. While it is generally safer to stick with plant-derived substances, we should not assume that because something comes from a plant, it can be used willy-nilly as an aphrodisiac.

The challenge is that some of the side-effects of long-term usage, may not be so obvious and vary between users. One way to test is that if you smoke marijuana regularly and you *only* get horny when you are smoking (and not at other times), you may be experiencing reduced dopamine intake through *'blunting'* of the dopamine receptors.[18] There is plenty of medical research into the positive and medicinal aspects of cannabis but, *caveat emptor*, long-term overuse might end up making you feel more flat, melancholic and lose your (sex) drive.

There is an easy test you can do to learn if your problem is due to reduced dopamine uptake. Stop smoking for a month or two and rate your daily mood and general horniness in a daily journal, from 0 to 10. This can help you notice any correlation between smoking and your general mood.

The good news is that blunting of the dopamine receptors is reversible. You will usually find that once the oil-based THC is completely out of your system, the receptors can repair themselves over a few (eg 4) weeks and your corresponding baseline horniness and happiness levels will usually return back to normal.

The bottom line is that shamanic crutches are only meant to be temporary. Ultimately, we all need to do the hard spiritual work to experience long-term personal and spiritual growth.

Photo credit: *Yung-pin Pao* (https://pixabay.com/users/jsbaw7160-828420/), https://pixabay.com/photos/oyster-shell-clams-dry-bay-seafood-989182/

---

18. https://www.psychologytoday.com/us/blog/the-athletes-way/201604/ heavy-marijuana-use-may-reduce-your-brains-dopamine-release

39

OUR SEX LIFE IS GREAT

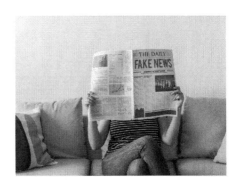

The Cost of Pretending

In a survey conducted by *iVillage*, 79% of the men thought their wives were either *'happy or very happy with their sex lives,'* but only 60 percent of the women said they actually were![1] The corollary is that pretending that our sex life is great does not make it so.

What is a *'great'* sex life, anyway? We can presume that the definition of *'great'* differs from one couple to the next, and also at various points in their life. 4 sexual interactions a week may be normal and desirable in your 30's, but when you are 50 with full-time jobs and kids to boot, having sex just once a week may be perfectly adequate. In fact, some studies show that people in relationship do not feel noticeably happier when they have sex more frequently than once a week.[2]

Whatever constitutes great sex for you, if you are not having it, pretending that all is good might be a way to ensure that it never will be. Honest (and often painful), acceptance of the truth is always the first step towards change. The energy and drive required to change usually come from accepting the painful reality that something is not how we want it to be.

---

1. https://www.today.com/health/ivillage-2013-married-sex-survey-results-1D80245229

2. Muise, Amy, Ulrich Schimmack, and Emily A. Impett. 'Sexual frequency predicts greater well-being, but more is not always better.' *Social Psychological and Personality Science* 7.4 (2016): 295-302.

Receiving Feedback

Men seem especially prone to having fragile sexual egos.[3] Nobody wants to think they are bad at sex, but if you are crap in bed, maybe it is time to bite the bullet and ask yourself *'why?'* For most people, being bad at sex is not a life sentence. More likely than not, this problem is fixable, but first you have to push past the pain of looking at the *'man in the mirror'*. If we see ourselves as being great in bed, acknowledging that we may have some things to learn in this department can be very upsetting to our self-image.

How often do we really ask for honest feedback on how we are doing in bed? It can be scary to ask that question if we are not prepared to accept a negative answer. In that case, it can be a lot easier to focus on specific actions. Instead of asking *'Do I suck in bed?'* you could ask something like *'What would you like more of in bed?'* That way, the feedback can be constructive and focused on behaviour rather than on your intrinsic self.

It seems exceptionally rare to find a man who is good in bed if they have not had any tantric training. Lack of variety, inability to circulate energy, repetitive movements, no-fuck talk and lack of empathy, make for mediocre friction-only-sex. The good news is that a real willingness to learn can quickly change all that. I mean in a few weeks. The tantra skills outlined in this book should be more than enough to give you a serious leg-up. Try them out and pay close attention to the other's responses during sex. That way you are using biofeedback to learn if your new skills are working or not.

Giving Feedback

What about the opposite situation? Do you have the skills to give delicate feedback and trust your partner enough to be honest with them? Are you afraid to deal with drama or retribution if you're totally honest? Here are some tips that might help:

- Ask permission first, to learn if they want feedback.
- Timing is everything. Patiently wait for a time when you both feel open, connected and relaxed.
- How we ask can make a big difference. Vulnerability, honesty, polite-

---

3. https://www.psypost.org/2017/03/
   men-view-womens-orgasms-masculinity-achievement-study-finds-48360

ness and genuine curiosity go a long way when it comes to offering suggestions on such a sensitive topic.

- Instead of the ultimate droop inducer *'You're crap in bed!'*, a more gentle approach with positive prompts such as *'I love it when you touch me slowly like that'* (even if he only does it one in a hundred times) may convey the same message with a much more enthusiastic uptake.

- Believe it or not, some people may find it easier to take in sensitive information more cleanly and logically if it is spelled out in written form in a clean way. Emailing on a sensitive subject can *sometimes* work better *if* it is done without emotional baggage, but sometimes this approach will backfire. It really seems to depend on the person and the topic.

Nevertheless, learning to convey information on vulnerable topics like sex can provide great communication tools that *'work like a charm'* in less volatile and more mundane areas of life.

Positive Thinking has Limits

The modern obsession with positive thinking can be useful in motivational situations, but new-age positive thinking can become quite toxic when it leads people to pretend that the reality is different from what the evidence suggests.[4] Positive thinking is rarely going to work in the bedroom. Thinking we are amazing sexual practitioners might fool ourselves temporarily, but it is hardly going to cut it for our partner.

Using the mind to try and rewrite reality may, in fact, halt personal growth. We need a certain amount of pain to drive change. If the stick part of the donkey-carrot setup is missing, we might not realise there is a problem, or be motivated to find and implement a solution. In other words, you can't think your problems away if those problems have practical implications.

With the popularity of social media and selfies, there is an allure to curate a happy-life image of ourselves that only includes happy faces. Every photo or post then becomes a means to seek self-validation and approval from our community. I am not a big social media fan. Why do so many people think that others will be interested in the details of their lives? Do

---

4. https://www.newstatesman.com/culture/2015/02/ happiness-conspiracy-against-optimism-and-cult-positive-thinking

they honestly think others are interested in seeing photos of their lunch on Facebook?[5,6] Is this caused by a subconscious longing to create envy in others? Do they think, *'I'm gonna eat this and you aren't?' 'Look at how successful I am!'* Isn't the obsession with *'me and my life'* just an ugly portrayal of ego in its most obnoxious form?

Regardless of the answers to these questions, one thing is certain, being fake is rarely sexy. Conversely, having depth and being real *are* sexy, and these qualities usually have their origins in taking a hard look at what could be improved.

Photo credit: *Rawpixel* (https://www.shutterstock.com/g/Rawpixel), https://www.shutterstock.com/image-photo/woman-reading-newspaper-1038686530

5. https://www.pewresearch.org/internet/fact-sheet/social-media/

6. https://www.socialmediatoday.com/social-networks/psychology-foodstagramming

40

SOME MEN ARE JUST BORN SEXIER THAN OTHERS

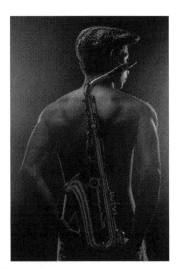

No. Much is Learnt Behaviour

What makes a man hot? Why do some men make our panties drop while others leave us cold? To really answer this question, let's examine the mechanics of masculine sex-appeal (and remember this can equally apply to masculine women). How much is hereditary, and how much is learnt behaviour that can be practised?

Courage

One of the sexiest things about a man is when he has the balls to *go the hard yard*. I don't just mean this in the traditional *machismo* sense, like swimming with sharks or wrestling with steers. What I am referring to is the internal fortitude to tackle difficult areas of his life and emotionally-charged situations. Is he able to confront his own fears and persist where others fail? Does he know his life's purpose and is he able to manifest it? Does he have the courage to stand by his convictions under fire? Does he walk-his-talk with integrity and honour?

When a man is manifesting his greatness despite adversity and fulfilling the dreams of his youth, now that is sexy! A man that has not compromised and sold out for security, comfort and mediocrity. A guy that stands for what he does and doesn't care so much about what others think or be so up-tight about his self-image. That is very sexy and very rare indeed.

Let's take an example dear to my heart. A lot of straight guys secretly are attracted to gender fluid people, but only the most confident have the gonads to sit in a restaurant with one.

There is no real reason in first world countries not to date a gender-fluid person other than caring about what others think. Hell, you can even be the head of state and be openly gay these days, as proven by the brave Elio Di Rupo.[1] It probably has more to do with the fear of being teased and joked about. But he only has to sit there and talk to me... I'm the one wearing the dress!

Abundance

I used to hate when people asked me what I do for a living, and I scoffed at women who appeared to be gold diggers surrounding successful guys. Now I get it. In fact now it is one of the first questions I ask. *'What do you do for a living?'* While there is not a 100% correlation, generally speaking, a guy with an interesting career and who has been successful, is *usually* more self-motivated, functional, confident and more likely to be interesting to talk to. Whether we admit it or not, success is often a female aphrodisiac. As a feminine person, it is easier to relax and be generous with my love, care and light in a beautiful environment, especially without financial stress. Who doesn't like to feel that they're hanging out with a winner?

Many women are attracted to successful men, but what exactly is success?[2] Money? Power? Prestige? When I was purely heterosexual, I thought the rationale behind it was that women wanted a good provider who could take care of them and their children. But now I can see that there is often something deeper going on when a woman is drawn to a successful man.[3,4] When a man is really great at something, especially when he excels in areas in which I'm weak, I admire his ability to apply sustained focus and drive to master his chosen field. He's competed out in the world and came out on

1. https://en.wikipedia.org/wiki/Elio_Di_Rupo

2. Townsend, J.M. & Levy, G.D. Arch Sex Behav (1990) 19: 149. https://doi.org/10.1007/BF01542229

3. https://www.psychologytoday.com/us/blog/the-attraction-doctor/201803/are-dominant-or-prestigious-men-more-attractive-women

4. Dunn, Michael J., and Alysia Hill. 'Manipulated luxury-apartment ownership enhances opposite-sex attraction in females but not males.' *Journal of Evolutionary Psychology* 12.1 (2014): 1-17.

top. He has proven he is capable of navigating his social environment in a way that is triumphant and perhaps capable of leading others at the same time... including me. If he knows more than I do about a particular area, then I can relax and let him have at it. It's sexy to look up to a man.

Even keel

Difficult situations and emotionally charged circumstances are brilliant testing grounds to measure masculinity. While one man may get hysterical, over-emotional and dramatic, another remains calm, collected and sees no point in taking it too seriously, which allows him to act more effectively. One of the biggest masculine gifts is being capable of zooming way out and putting things into a bigger context, while not getting lost in emotions, and frantically changing things in a knee-jerk reaction because they can't handle the discomfort. In traditional masculine meditation, the ability to feel through the appearance of the moment and into the underlying masculine essence of undivided consciousness is called *transcendence*. Staying level in rocky seas is a measure of being able to manifest and display this transcendent meditation in daily life, and crisis is the ultimate testing ground to see what men are really made of.

Humour

I don't mean who knows the best jokes (although that can be kind of sexy). By humour, I'm talking about the type of guy who can laugh at himself and dust himself off after a fall, and then get back in the saddle with a smile. The definition of a joke is leading someone down a corridor of logic and then unexpectedly turning left when everyone thinks they know things are going straight ahead. For example, the old joke where a guy comes into the pub with a big smile on his face, announcing to his buddies that he had his first blowjob, to which one of his friends retorts with, *'Well then can you please rinse your mouth out before sharing my glass!'*. Being able to zoom right back and detach from the situation is more of a masculine trait. Have you ever wondered why so many female tennis stars and comedians are lesbians or women with dominant masculine sides?

Humour is often mentioned in men's online dating profiles: *'Loves sushi, down-to-earth and has a good sense of humour.'* What the feminine often values about quick wit is that it's a manifestation of being intelligent, undramatic and relaxed rather than *'Oh he's so funny! I bet he's great in bed and a good provider!'*

Discipline

Self-discipline in a man is sexy because it shows he can tough it out when needed. One of the traditional methods common to many masculine spiritual practices is renunciation and abstinence, and giving up sex can be one of the most difficult discipline practices. But there is a problem with *traditional* abstinence practices, in that they don't seem to be sustainable except for asexual people, and studies show that only about 1%-1.7% of the population identify as asexual.[5,6] For the rest of us, abstinence usually leads to sexual suppression. Finding a modern way of renunciation such as avoiding the instant gratification of the pudendal-nerve orgasm *while* staying sexually active may be a useful test of a man's strength of resolve and discipline. It appears this practice may be more difficult for men because they have to master the use of their pudendal nerve (penis) during sex to satisfy another.

Muscles?

Focusing on abs, pecs and glutes seems rather superficial, but there may be deeper reasons for this attraction. From an evolutionary perspective, health and attraction go hand in hand. Statistically, women are more likely to be attracted to tall men who have a muscular upper body and a narrow waist, with the implication being that they make better breeding stock.[7] This is just another variable that is in the man's control.

Attractiveness

For men, there is some value in being conventionally attractive. As far as the face goes, in general, women prefer a man with a symmetrical face, a wide jaw and average size facial features.[8] However, this factor is less im-

---

5. Anthony F. Bogaert (2004) Asexuality: Prevalence and associated factors in a national probability sample, *The Journal of Sex Research*, 41:3, 279-287, DOI: 10.1080/00224490409552235

6. https://williamsinstitute.law.ucla.edu/press/press-releases/asexual-lgb-press-release/

7. https://www.psychologytoday.com/us/blog/cutting-edge-leadership/201207/which-body-shapes-are-most-sexually-attractive

8. https://www.psychologytoday.com/us/blog/cutting-edge-leadership/201206/what-does-the-shape-your-face-say-about-you

portant to women than it is to men. In a 2015 study by social scientists at Chapman University, 84 percent of the women said that *'It was 'desirable/ essential' that their potential partner was good-looking'* as compared with 92 percent of men.[9]

Confidence

Confidence is, perhaps, the ultimate turn-on. It can't be faked easily, but is something hard-won through living successfully, upbringing and mastering a chosen career. Sorry, no short-cuts on this one.

Finally

Very few of us are born with Brad Pitt's charm and quirky, cute smile, or with George Clooney's charisma and chiselled jaw. The good thing about the deeper aspects of masculine attractiveness is that most of them are behavioural and can be learned and developed... and often get better with age! So guys, not many viable victim excuses here! The ball's in your court.

Photo credit: *Aaron Cabrera* (https://pixabay.com/users/aaron00023-790223/), https://pixabay.com/photos/music-musician-concert-band-3264711/

---

9.   https://www.eurekalert.org/pub_releases/2015-09/cu-cup091615.php

41

MEN OVER FOCUS ON LOOKS

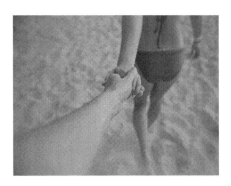

Are looks That Important?

Among many others, a 2006 study from Rice University, indicates that conventionally attractive people are given more breaks in life. As unfair as it seems, both sexes trust beautiful people more. We are more likely to give them a job, and usually pay them better salaries.[1] We do this because we are programmed to assume they are smarter and more trustworthy than ordinary people.[2] This phenomenon is known as the halo effect.[3] Just go into any club during the weekend and you will undoubtedly see that people with movie-star looks are often treated preferentially, particularly in the club scene, because other people are more interested in having sex with them.[4]

Whose Issue is it?

Arguably, Western culture has deeply ingrained beauty standards that drive many young women to eating disorders, low self-esteem and de-

---

1. https://www.businessinsider.com/
   attractive-people-are-more-successful-2012-9?r=US&IR=T

2. http://news.rice.edu/2006/09/21/
   rice-study-suggests-people-are-more-trusting-of-attractive-strangers/

3. https://www.psychologytoday.com/gb/basics/the-halo-effect

4. https://www.psychologytoday.com/gb/blog/games-primates-play/201203/
   the-truth-about-why-beautiful-people-are-more-successful

pression.[5] Everywhere we look, photoshopped images of slender, glossy haired, able-bodied women represent the Hollywood beauty standard.[6] These highly-edited images of people (especially women) have become ubiquitous in our lives due to widespread access of photo editing tools on people's phones.[7] There are representations of this type of beauty in virtually every movie, TV show, video game and online ad. The beauty industry pours billions of dollars every year into cosmetic aids in the knowledge that many of us will fork out money to try and live up to those standards. This has become so pervasive that countries are pushing back by banning excessively-retouched images in advertising.[8]

As a consequence, it should come as no surprise that many feminine women spend a lot of time obsessing about their looks[9] and comparing themselves unfavourably to celebrities and sexual rivals in their community.[10,11] To the surprise of many men, female competition is just as cutthroat as in the men's arena.

Different Genders have Different Attractors

We've all seen couples that appear to be mismatched in the physical beauty department, right? A woman with a perfect hourglass figure and dressed to kill, with a man who is nowhere near as hot. He's balding and his clothes don't fit him well, but his Rolex and nice car seem to be more than making up for it. Women are not necessarily less superficial than men, they are

5. https://www.psychologytoday.com/gb/blog/media-spotlight/201311/media-exposure-and-the-perfect-body

6. https://www.psychologytoday.com/us/blog/when-food-is-family/201404/culture-dictates-the-standard-beauty

7. https://www.theguardian.com/media/2018/mar/09/facetune-photoshopping-app-instagram-body-image-debate

8. https://www.telegraph.co.uk/news/politics/liberaldemocrats/6516537/Airbrushed-images-harming-girls-and-boys-experts-say.html

9. https://www.telegraph.co.uk/news/uknews/6634686/Women-worry-about-their-bodies-252-times-a-week.html

10. https://www.psychologytoday.com/us/blog/beauty-sick/201804/why-you-cant-stop-comparing-yourself-media-images

11. https://www.psychologytoday.com/gb/blog/insight-therapy/201401/feminine-foes-new-science-explores-female-competition

just looking for different things.[12] As we discussed in the previous chapter, the feminine is primed to look for indicators that the man is successful, confident and can provide a level of abundance. Personally, I notice a pronounced shift in focus when switching from male to female personas. When I'm in my male role, I'm much more concerned with career than with how physically attractive I appear... and vice versa in femme mode.

The thought that 'looks are not important' may be more of a female reaction to try and pacify obsessive feminine thinking. Let me explain. The hilarious YouTube video 'Hot and Crazy/Cute and Money matrix' makes fun of gender disparities in our society.[13] Men not being as highly prized for beauty as women are, and success appealing more to women than to men, makes for a very politically-incorrect laugh.

Of course, no generalisation is true for every individual, but broad patterns that point out the difference between genders can be quite illuminating. For example, as a workshop facilitator, I have the opportunity to survey many women on this topic. I have frequently asked how often women hear the voice of feminine self-concern when they sit idly, doing nothing. I was surprised to hear that preoccupation with looks and relationship fills about 75% of their idle thinking time. Compare that to the response of men who say they are thinking about their looks and relationship about 5-10% of their idle thinking time. Men's passive thinking seems to revolve more around sex, career, planning and problem-solving.

At the start of their personal development, many women think that worrying about their looks is superficial, believing that plastic surgery, make-up or even attractive clothing are 'un-spiritual'.[14] I used to think that too. The problem with this stance is that, when you analyse it, it reveals a self-centred way of thinking. We are not the ones who have to look at ourselves! Would we really want to walk down the street and see everyone dressed like a bum? Don't you enjoy seeing beauty in the world around you? In a way, isn't it a gift to others to look attractive and make the world a tiny bit more visually-pleasing by being well-dressed and groomed?

Following this train of thought, what is the difference between clothing

---

12. https://www.psychologytoday.com/gb/blog/talking-apes/201907/do-women-really-prefer-men-money-over-looks

13. https://www.youtube.com/watch?v=incSwssUyp4

14. https://www.theguardian.com/commentisfree/2016/jan/25/appearance-secret-life-beauty-receptionist

and the physical body, aesthetically speaking? Personally, I'm all for plastic surgery, even though such a statement can raise a few eyebrows due to the social stigma around cosmetic body modifications. Look at how many Hollywood actors deny having had plastic surgery.[15,16] Whether they did it or not, they feel offended when people ask, and feel the need to refute such claims because people often shame others about getting plastic surgery for purely cosmetic reasons.[17]

Millennials seem to be more relaxed in this area than older generations. In a study done by the American Academy of Facial Plastic and Reconstructive Surgery (AAFPRS), *72% of facial plastic surgeons have noticed an increase of patients under 30 years old.*[18] Perhaps the stigma about plastic surgery is heading in the direction of the dodo bird, as it well should! Maybe then, people will feel more free to do whatever they choose with their bodies.

Of course, accepting yourself as you are is a good thing. That's step 1. Step 2 is asking yourself, *'How can I serve the world better with my physical appearance?'* If it makes you feel more confident and your partner likes it, why *not* get your boobs done? Why not pin back protruding ears, get laser treatment on a noticeable birthmark or change the shape of your nose—like Lisa Kudrow did—if you think it will make you happier about your looks?[19] Why not take a class and learn how to master your make-up for the sake of gifting your beauty to the world?

Not caring about looks certainly makes it more difficult to strike a good first impression,[20] so why make life harder for you than it has to be? As an added bonus, some researchers believe that wearing make-up has positive psychological effects. Make-up can make some women feel prettier and

---

15. https://people.com/celebrity/stars-denying-plastic-surgery-rumors/

16. https://www.nickiswift.com/3894/celebs-spent-plastic-surgery/

17. https://www.huffingtonpost.co.uk/antonia-mariconda/cosmetic-surgery-shaming_b_9877192.html

18. https://www.americanspa.com/medical-spa/study-reveals-increase-millennial-patients-opting-plastic-surgery

19. https://www.elle.com/beauty/health-fitness/a26805/why-do-we-shame-women-who-get-plastic-surgery/

20. https://www.psychologytoday.com/us/blog/wander-woman/201107/why-women-have-care-about-their-looks

more self-confident.[21] One study even suggests it makes women smarter![22] My advice is to do the best you can before you go out and, as you walk out the door, try to place less attention on yourself and ignore your inner critic as much as possible by focusing on your partner. Of course, the practice of focusing more on others than ourselves is beneficial for everyone, regardless of gender.

While men may be attracted to women who meet their aesthetic taste, on a deeper level they are looking for women who are confident in their sexiness and who are open, generous with their love, positive and happy, as physical appearance only goes so far. This is something you may know from meeting someone who you regarded as super-attractive, right until they opened their pretty mouth and started spewing out garbage.[23,24] Unlike age, most of these variables listed above *are* under our control.

Photo credit: *Stokpic* (https://pixabay.com/users/stokpic-692575/), https://pixabay.com/photos/couple-beach-holding-hands-bikini-677585/

21. https://www.nytimes.com/roomfordebate/2013/01/02/does-makeup-hurt-self-esteem/ makeup-can-provide-a-fleeting-confidence-boost-to-some

22. Rocco Palumbo, Beth Fairfield, Nicola Mammarella & Alberto Di Domenico | Peter Walla (Reviewing Editor) (2017) Does make-up make you feel smarter? The 'lipstick effect' extended to academic achievement, *Cogent Psychology*, 4:1, DOI: 10.1080/23311908.2017.1327635

23. https://www.psychologytoday.com/gb/blog/the-attraction-doctor/201105/ is-your-personality-making-you-more-or-less-physically-attractive

24. http://www.spsp.org/news-center/blog/romanticconfidence

42

HE LOVES MY LINGERIE

Maybe not...

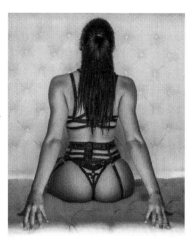

Let me be clear from the start. I believe that everybody has the right to decide what makes them feel sexy and to wear whatever they damn well please. Some feminine people like to use sexy underwear for an evening alone, pampering themselves and focusing on their self-care. Others enjoy wearing something naughty under their clothes at work while looking perfectly square on the outside. If you enjoy wearing lingerie only for *yourself*, then it makes sense to choose your lingerie with only your pleasure in mind.

However...

Ladies, have you ever had the experience of dressing up in sexy lingerie and feeling that positive response from your male partner is a little forced and somewhat lacking in enthusiasm? There might be a very good reason for this. Men and women have very different ideas on what classifies as *'sexy'* when it comes to lingerie, and they rarely seem to communicate that to each other.[1] Many men secretly confess their frustration on this subject to me, so I thought I would share it with my sisters and devote an entire chapter on the subject. In the name of not wasting precious money on something that you love and he is pretty *'meh'* about, it might be worth investing some time in finding out what lingerie men really find sexy, if you are interested in making your man more attracted to you that is.

---

1.   https://betches.com/what-guys-really-think-of-lingerie/

Different Strokes for Different Folks

Unless you are in the habit of communicating with radical honesty, chances are that he may be actually withholding his lacklustre feelings about your lingerie simply because he doesn't want to offend you and risk forced sexual abstinence (see the next chapter for more on this topic). Most predominantly masculine people will often swallow their words to avoid risking confrontation and drama. So if you really want to nail the correct attire you might have to coax out of him what he really likes.

Walking through a mall, most lingerie shops seem crammed with multi-colour, lacey, flowery items for women to buy. Oftentimes, these are the last thing men would consider sexy, though they will rarely admit it. If you have a super-sweet, nice-guy partner that tries to please you all the time, he will probably set aside his own specific desires and try to buy you something he predicts you will like, usually in the more sweet-and-innocent end of the spectrum.[2] The corollary is that his birthday gift to you may not actually reflect what kind of lingerie he finds sexy. Yet lingerie can have a huge impact on a man's level of attraction to you.[3] Expecting what you wear to be irrelevant does not make it so. Men are typically aroused more visually than women, so a woman's physical appearance is important to a man.[4] Pretending otherwise for the sake of political correctness is just denying reality.

I'm not suggesting you only wear the clothes and lingerie that your man wants you to wear like an obedient pet. What I'm talking about is making small sacrifices in comfort out of strength, to give him the gift of what probably is the most valuable thing to him, your sexual beauty adorned as an offering... to his taste.

Research

So, how do you learn what he really likes? One way of coaxing this information out of him can be inviting him to look at lingerie with you. That shouldn't be so difficult! Ask him to point out what lingerie he's most attracted to. Tell him not to worry about your modesty or taste because

2. https://www.psychologytoday.com/us/blog/all-about-sex/201402/valentines-day-mans-guide-buying-lingerie-women

3. http://fashionispsychology.com/the-psychology-of-lingerie/

4. https://www.sciencedaily.com/releases/2004/03/040316072953.htm

you want to push your own boundaries. You might be shocked to find that what he chooses is a lot sluttier than you expected. If you don't believe me, do some market research of your own. Go into a strip club and see what the professionals wear. Feel free to take a card out of the playbook of the women who conduct extensive market surveys of men, every night. Their ability to feed themselves depends on getting it right.

A Few Pointers

- Women seem to like wearing flowers, but this is a big turn off for most men. My advice is to back away slowly from the flower selection unless you have a horny horticulturist husband or roleplaying the sweet-girl turnaround.

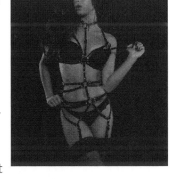

- Another common feminine mistake is multi-colour lingerie. Stick with one colour girls! Mainly black or occasionally red or another darker colour, for variety. White satin (not cotton) can also be useful to achieve a virginal look. Whatever you choose, the rule here is keeping things minimal rather than complex.
- Men usually prefer much simpler lingerie than women. Simple, good quality, French lingerie is often at the top of most men's taste.
- Lace is a rather mixed bag. Some love it and some hate it, but one thing to take into account is that lace is not as enjoyable to the touch as silk or satin. Actually, it can feel like a cheese-grater under the hand, when you stroke it. It's usually best to keep it to a minimum, unless he specifically likes it.
- Silk or satin seems to be a no-brainer. For the more adventurous; vinyl, latex or leather.
- Most men love straight lines against flesh. Hence, thigh-high stockings and suspenders are always a big hit. I very rarely hear a man that doesn't like them.

- For hard-to-find slutty items, find out where strippers buy their lingerie. Remember, those girls have done much of the market research in the dark end of the feminine spectrum for you.
- Variety is valuable. If you want to embody a lot of different flavours of the feminine, it can be useful to have sexy lingerie that helps you to alternate between looking and feeling whatever

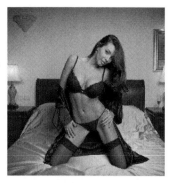

flavours you are channelling, such as the virgin, the mother, the sacred whore, etc.

Why Compromise?

What if I'm right and you find that the lingerie that he likes is outside of your comfort zone? Then you have a choice to make. It's totally reasonable to choose to remain in your comfort zone. Alternatively, you could use this information as a potential opportunity to expand your boundaries and continue the process of overcoming your internal slut shaming mechanism. Yes, you might look like a sex worker... but so what?

Please don't get me wrong after reading this chapter in thinking that I'm saying "ALL flowery, lacy and non-black lingerie" looks ugly and unappealing to ALL men. No, there certainly are many men who love these flavours as well (the bimbo look, etc.). But the point I'm trying to bring across is that the flavour of "hard" slut or whore energy is typically underused by women and their men may be starving for that look in particular.

The average virile male usually has a sizeable appetite for the naughty girl, so it pays to supply that longing yourself with a stable diet of weekly dark sexual energy, because if you're not interested in providing it, then you might discover that he seeks it out elsewhere. If he feels guilty because he likes the dark, slutty end of the feminine spectrum and you are the one denying him access to it, this may cause a slow, choking death of your sexual relationship. Shaming him into pretending he doesn't like what he does may ultimately teach him to compromise and act contrary to his nature. Do you find men that do that sexy?

For all of us, personal growth is maturing from seeking to serving, and there seem to be few areas where that switch can be so immediately and tangibly practised as it can in this hidden domain.

43

SEX IS A REWARD

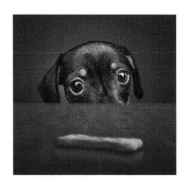

But Can Also Be a Weapon

In my estimation, 99% of heterosexual men in a monogamous relationship have avoided doing or saying something for fear of being denied sex by their partner. If you noticed that your lover is upset and that it equates to being confined to the *'no-sex tonight couch'*, this may lead to the habit of avoiding confrontation to ensure uninterrupted access to sex. While virtually all couples do this, there is a hidden cost that most seem unaware of: the loss of mutual sexual attraction.

I used to believe that harmony was the best outcome. Being right just wasn't worth the battle and I would rather just move on and *'fuggedaboudit'*. However, after analysing this situation further, I realised that caving-in only succeeded in creating a short-term harmony. In the long-run, acquiescence is the silent killer of sexual attraction because it breeds passive aggression and resentment, and reinforces the notion that manipulation actually works. Many *'overly soft'* men confess to giving up boundaries too easily because of the risk of being labelled a *'macho jerk'* or *'insensitive to women's values'.* These labels are some of the worst perceived insults for *'nice guys'*.

While micro-managing and over-controlling a man (which is all too common in 1st world countries) can create a very compliant sweet guy, the problem is that women are rarely attracted to neutered men. When a woman withholds sex to control a man's behaviour (a practice that is colloquially referred to as *pussy-whipping*), this commonly creates the opposite of the desired effect. Relaxed confidence in a man is sexy; a tepid boy asking questions because he doesn't want to do something wrong, is not.[1]

What Is the Solution?

In my experience, feminine people often avoid sex after an argument. (Now is probably a good time to repeat that I'm using the word *'feminine'* and not *'female'*. Both sexes can go into destructive feminine patterns). For men, hoping for harmony to happen by endlessly discussing a subject may be paramount to driving a McLaren 720s and being stuck in first gear. An alternative and more efficient route to reconnect after a struggle is called *'fuck first, talk second!'* The outcome is you usually won't have so much to talk about afterwards and the disagreement may seem trivial in the afterglow of good sex.[2] There is plenty of evidence that emotional distance between partners can be alleviated by a nice dose of oxytocin.[3] A certain magic can happen when we drop our mental stories and let our bodies initiate the healing. Trying to talk a loggerhead situation to its resolution can be a needlessly tedious endeavour.

Specific Skills

The New Tantra has an extensive workshop on how to lovingly help a feminine person (man or woman) escape destructive feminine patterns such as drama (and we have identified more than 25 of those patterns).[4] The key is to avoid the common mistakes of getting angry or turning into soppy conforming wimps.

During my first delivery of this workshop, I was rather shocked to find out just how inexperienced men were at supporting women effectively out of their destructive negative patterns of behaviour. I've never seen a man able to deal with more than one of the 25 destructive patterns successfully! It seems that men have very little innate understanding of how to lovingly help someone navigate through their intense emotions. Needless to say, it's a useful workshop!

Bottom line: never use sex as a weapon to force someone to obey your

---

1.   https://www.goodtherapy.org/blog/women-committed-relationships-lose-sexual-desire/

2.   https://www.psychologytoday.com/us/blog/dating-decisions/201506/the-truth-about-make-sex

3.   https://www.medicalnewstoday.com/articles/275795.php

4.   TNT Men's Workshop. https://www.thenewtantra.com/

will. The problem is that even if you win, you lose. If a woman does it to a man, he'll probably end up resentful and distant and she'll unknowingly put herself in the position of a mommy, thus losing the respect and attraction to him in the process.

Photo credit: *Johan Swanepoel* (https://www.shutterstock.com/g/johan63), https://www.shutterstock.com/image-photo/dachshund-puppy-looking-treat-out-reach-366838454

44

BDSM IS A PERVERSION

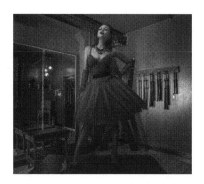

Feminine Longing to Surrender

Let's start this chapter with a little confession. I was a severe life-experi-ence-box-checker. I had a terminal case of FOMO (fear of missing out.) I started out with superficial things like travelling to 46 countries, cars, adrenaline sports, etc., but ended up seeking experiences capable of ex-panding my understanding of life and the world we live in.[1] Better to do too much than too little. I'd rather waste a little time finding that it wasn't worth it than regret not having tried something and missing the boat.[2] As a result, I have experienced more than most people, especially in the realm of sexuality. Many things I didn't expect to find interesting proved to be rather eye-opening, and some of those eventually became part of my stable sexual diet. I found most of those alternatives on the other side of my conditioned fears, judgements and resistances.

Consider for example BDSM. This acronym stands for *'a combination of the abbreviations B/D (bondage and discipline), D/S (dominance and sub-mission), and S/M (sadism and masochism).'*[3,4] Although I have no judgment about those who enjoy the darkest end of the BDSM spectrum, my per-

1. https://www.psychologytoday.com/us/blog/inviting-monkey-tea/201809/
    are-you-tired-chasing-amazing-experiences

2. https://medium.com/the-mission/
    to-overcome-the-fear-of-failure-fear-this-instead-d880ce3e5ccf

3. Luo, Siyang, and Xiao Zhang. 'Embodiment and Humiliation Moderation of Neural Responses to Others' Suffering in Female Submissive BDSM Practitioners.' *Frontiers in neuroscience* 12 (2018): 463.

4. https://www.psychologytoday.com/us/blog/the-compass-pleasure/201503/
    the-neurobiology-bdsm-sexual-practice

sonal taste is for the more subtle and tantric end of this smorgasbord... and yes I have been shown the ropes (so to speak) by some of Europe's best.

Healthy BDSM

I doubt many book publishers were *not* shocked by the phenomenal success of *'Fifty Shades of Grey.'*[5] It certainly leveraged a huge untapped market of female longing.[6] BDSM may not be all about pleasure-seeking. There is evidence that BDSM has many positive aspects in other parts of life. For instance, in a study published in 2013, Dutch scientists found that *'BDSM practitioners were less neurotic, more extraverted, more open to new experiences, more conscientious, less rejection sensitive, [and] had higher subjective well-being,'* as compared with a control group of non-BDSM practitioners.[7] Another study published by Dr Pamela H. Connolly in 2008, suggests that BDSM practitioners don't experience the negative effects that many people imagine from dark role-plays. Depression, anxiety and post-traumatic stress disorder (PTSD) were not found at any higher rates than in non-BDSM practitioners. Another study by Dr Brad Sagarin, creator of The Science of BDSM website,[8] found that after BDSM play, both dominant and submissive partners felt closer and less stressed than before the play.[9,10]

Leading

Learning how to lead with authority, logic, emotional intelligence and intuition is a very useful masculine skill (for both men and women).[11] It requires feeling into the other person and knowing what they long for but are reluctant to ask for. Learning how to communicate verbally and nonverbally, and

---

5. Wismeijer, Andreas AJ, and Marcel ALM Van Assen. 'Psychological characteristics of BDSM practitioners.' *The Journal of Sexual Medicine* 10.8 (2013): 1943-1952.

6. https://www.lehmiller.com/blog/2015/2/6/why-fifty-shades-of-grey-is-not-a-how-to-guide-for-bdsm

7. https://www.ncbi.nlm.nih.gov/pubmed/23679066

8. http://www.scienceofbdsm.com/

9. https://www.ncbi.nlm.nih.gov/pubmed/18563549

10. https://www.theguardian.com/commentisfree/2015/feb/09/bdsm-good-for-you-fifty-shades-of-grey-relationship

11. Pliskin, Eli. 'Social and Emotional Intelligence (SEI) in BDSM.' *Journal of Positive Sexuality* 4.2 (2018).

getting explicit consent[12] about what the other person wants is necessary to be able to perceive someone else's limits and boundaries, even if they are tied up with a ball gag in their mouth!

Masculinity is often measured in someone's skill at leading. The next time you hear her cry *'Why can't you be more masculine!'* She may be simply longing to not have to lead you. Can there be a more unmistakable way to learn the art of leading than in such a polarised situation?

Surrendering

Conversely, learning how to follow and surrender is a very useful (and arousing) feminine skill (again, applicable to both men and women). Some people struggle because they always feel the impetus to control the situation, even when they are meant to be surrendering.[13] In BDSM, this behaviour is called *'topping from the bottom'*.[14]

In the bedroom, there is something inherently sexy about surrendering to someone who is good at leading. Their desire for you can simply be shown through action by pulling you close, deciding which direction you should face or telling you what to expect next. For someone who has to be constantly in control in their everyday life, not having to use their masculine decision-making mind and allowing themselves to be directed can be heaven in itself and highly arousing, even without taking off the clothes.

Switching

The best surrendering often comes from strong leaders. Always being in the driver's seat is very limiting. It limits your perspective, which is why the best *'tops'* have often *'bottomed'* and those best at domination have spent significant time being dominated. You learn empathy by taking on the opposite role.

Many strong, successful people often confess to routinely visiting BDSM clubs or dominatrixes. They happily spend loads of money to take on the submissive role in a sexual interaction. And, why not! It can be like

---

12. https://medium.com/@themicheab/can-bdsm-teach-us-what-were-missing-on-consent-and-bodily-autonomy-581c2cf4433f

13. https://boldpleasures.com/kinky-life/ditch-shame/alpha-subs-letting-go/

14. https://www.bustle.com/p/what-does-christian-say-at-the-end-of-fifty-shades-freed-the-line-ends-the-franchise-on-a-sexy-note-8161886

an intense vacation from the role as chief fire-suppressor.

Power play, bondage, light spanking, cross-dressing, fetish clothing and role-playing can all be a fun part of sexual play. It's also a great reminder not to take ourselves too seriously or a way to take our minds completely off a busy day at the office. I mean, if you can think about doing your end-of-year accounts or the latest stock prices whilst in 8 inch heels doing a catwalk for your mistress, it's probably not the deepest mind-blowing session you're having!

Caution

Where BDSM may have an unhealthy psychological side is when it capitalises on past childhood trauma by replaying it endlessly for sexual gratification. This tends to happen when the individual is not consciously choosing to re-enact the scene with the purpose of healing but to act it out compulsively for kicks.[15] This is where people might need to be careful. Continually re-enacting something traumatic to try and clear the situation could simply be an addiction and *getting off on it* usually does not lead anywhere useful, unless it includes some aftercare in which the trauma can be processed in a safe environment.[16] The masochistic embrace of humiliation, excessive pain and damaging the body sometimes reflects a degree of self-hatred. However, even in these situations, there is some suggestion that BDSM can be used as a method for harm-reduction.[17] More studies are needed in this highly sensitive area.

Photo credit: *Alexandr Ivanov* (https://pixabay.com/users/ivanovgood-1982503/), https://wallpapers.io/photo/6996-bdsm-red-woman-wallpaper

---

15. https://www.psychologytoday.com/us/blog/understanding-the-erotic-code/201502/shades-play-trauma-reenactment-versus-trauma-play

16. https://www.psychologytoday.com/us/blog/standard-deviations/201805/growing-kinky-research-shows-how-kink-identity-is-formed

17. https://www.psychologytoday.com/us/blog/standard-deviations/201610/bdsm-harm-reduction

45

WET DREAMS ARE UNCONTROLLABLE
Dream Yoga

Nocturnal emissions, colloquially known as wet dreams, appear to be uncontrollable since they happen in an unconscious dream state. Most articles reviewed by medical professionals admit that they are impossible to control fully. However, they do provide some suggestions for behavioural modifications you can try, while also acknowledging their lack of effectiveness.[1,2] Apparently, we are victims of our subconscious minds. In the words of the famous psychoanalyst Carl Gustav Jung, *Until you make the unconscious conscious, it will direct your life and you will call it fate.* But this is an area where tantra *can* help. Many men notice that their wet dreams stop once they understand why they are happening and adjust their lifestyle accordingly. Here is how it works:

Remember Your Dreams

Your first step is to figure out what you are dreaming about when you have a nocturnal emission. Moving the fantasy from the subconscious to the conscious mind may help stop it from happening in the dream. Pay attention to your dreams and try to remember as many details as possible. Keep a journal on your bed-side table and write what happened in the dream as soon as you wake up. What was the sexual situation or scenario

---

1. https://www.medicalnewstoday.com/articles/321351.php#prevention
2. https://www.healthline.com/health/healthy-sex/wet-dreams#prevention

you were dreaming about? Were there any other factors that you can see a pattern of?[3] Is it something that excites you but you haven't done in real life? If it is, it may be that your subconscious is trying to fulfil this desire by acting it out in your dream. Sigmund Freud and Carl Jung both believed that *'Dreams can reveal a person's deepest unconscious wishes and desires.'*[4] For example, dreaming about having sex with a person of the same gender may be a way for your unconscious-self to scratch that itch for you without the shame of doing it in real life.

For the brave, though, there is another option. Just as we mentioned before with masturbation fantasies, identify what you are longing for and consciously act it out tantrically in real life with (an) other consenting adult(s). There are different ways to go about this, but one safe way may be to begin exploring any sex-positive or conscious sex communities around you.[5] Sex-positive people have, by definition, positive attitudes and open minds about sex and they are usually comfortable with most (safe, sane and consensual) sexual situations. Depending on where you live, you might find that you have to travel quite far away to find one, but if you are in a metropolitan area it may be as easy as looking on *Meetup* or browsing for sex-positive groups on social media to find a suitable sex-positive event.[6,7] Once you have met a few compatible people who you trust and feel safe with, you can begin a conversation about acting out your dream in real life.

In my experience teaching this technique, liberating this desire from the subconscious to the conscious mind stops the wet dreams from happening in 8 out of 10 men. Unfortunately, it's not a sure-fire cure, but there is one last method.

While I don't think it is healthy to become too religious about the no-cumming thing, it can be quite satisfying to know that you have mastered it for some time... including when you are asleep. I found the only way to completely stop the wet dreams was to really notice (and even exaggerate) the negative effects of ejaculation when they happened. I used to vent my exasperation out loud, with a lot of emotion when I had a *'miss'*

3. https://www.metromaleclinic.com/night-fall-in-men-wet-dreams/
4. https://www.psychologytoday.com/us/blog/out-the-ooze/201801/the-freudian-symbolism-in-your-dreams
5. https://www.issm.info/sexual-health-qa/what-does-sex-positive-mean/
6. https://www.meetup.com/topics/sex-positive/
7. https://thecspc.org/event

so that my subconscious could hear it. That clear verbal communication of disappointment was the driving force that got through to my subconscious and would even set off alarm bells in the middle of a dream when I got into dangerously horny situations. Only then did my wet dreams totally cease to happen. Your mileage may vary.

Photo credit: *Matthew Hyatt* (https://www.shutterstock.com/g/matthew+hyatt), https://www.shutterstock.com/image-photo/water-ripples-633990632

46

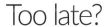

SEX EDUCATION SHOULD START AT PUBERTY

Too late?

It should come as no surprise that most adults have a lot of unconscious shame around sex[1] which can lead to any number of knock-on-effects in relationships.[2] This sexual shame often makes it difficult to talk about sex with others, and there is much evidence that this can ruin long-term sexual relationships, as well as be passed along from generation to generation.

Sex Education from Parents

A female friend of mine was raised in a conservative religious family. When her school sent her home with a book on sex education to be read with her parents, they were so embarrassed that they kept making jokes when reading the text. So, when she became exasperated and turned to leave the room, they just told her, *'Well, we think you know what we expect of you.'* Was this their way of telling her that abstinence and sex within marriage were the only acceptable choices for her? In this same family, her mother never spoke to her about menstruation, but rather threw a pamphlet and a single pad onto her bed when she was 10 and then walked away, never to mention it again. When she started masturbating, she didn't even know

---

1. https://www.goodtherapy.org/blog/is-shame-affecting-your-sex-life-0830185
2. https://health.howstuffworks.com/sexual-health/sexual-dysfunction/sexual-guilt-and-shame-dictionary.htm

what it was called. She would press her vulva against her pillows and when her genital area started throbbing she became afraid, thinking she was going to die. She got numerous yeast infections during her teenage years and they all went untreated because she could not bring herself to tell her parents about the itching *'down there.'*[3,4]

That's a pretty extreme example of sex-shame parenting, but even liberal, open-minded parents that think they don't have much sexual shame may be unconsciously sending strong shame signals to their children. An example I heard many times is *'My children can ask me any questions about sex, however they just don't seem to bring up the subject... but they shouldn't be shy.'* Children learn by example, so if their parents act coy around the subject of sex and never mention it in a relaxed and comfortable way then, what chance does the child have of transcending their parents' shame and spontaneously broaching the topic of sex?

Young people do not wake up on their thirteenth birthday, somehow transformed into a sexual being overnight. Even young children are sexual in some form. —Heather Coleman, PhD & Grant Charles, PhD University of Calgary, Alberta, Canada, and The University of British Columbia, Vancouver.[5]

So why then do parents so often believe that children don't have sexual feelings? Starting from inside the womb, foetuses and young children try to touch their genitalia because it feels good.[6] As they get older, their sexuality is expressed through sexual behaviour, some of which they do privately, making it easier for parents to pretend their children don't have sexual feelings.[7,8]

Sadly, there are still many squeamish parents who can't or won't talk to their children about sex. Some parents will not permit their children to get sex education in school for fear that it will encourage them to be

---

3. https://www.vice.com/en_us/article/pa98x8/purity-culture-linday-kay-klein-pure-review
4. https://www.psychologytoday.com/us/blog/women-who-stray/201708/overcoming-religious-sexual-shame
5. Coleman, H., & Charles, G. (2001). Adolescent sexuality: A matter of condom sense. *Journal of Child and Youth Care*, 14 (4), 17-18.
6. https://www.nytimes.com/2018/12/10/well/family/why-is-childrens-masturbation-such-a-secret.html
7. https://www.kidshealth.org.nz/sexual-behaviour-children-and-young-people
8. Kellogg, Nancy D. 'Sexual behaviors in children: Evaluation and management.' *American Family Physician* 82.10 (2010): 1233.

promiscuous. That's *not* how it works, of course. Instead, we end up with a generation of children who are undereducated or ashamed to talk about what actually happens in sex.

It seems that many parents procrastinate on this subject not just because it is uncomfortable but also due to the complexity of the subject and how much information is too much information. Sex education is not just about learning to put on a condom or saying no to sex. You wouldn't expect to give your kid a tutu and send them off to an audition for Swan Lake. But then, what should they speak about and what feels *'too grown up for them, right now?'* When is the right time to talk about sexual orientation, gender expression, consent and communication, pleasure and sensitivity, body positivity, safer sex and sexually transmitted infections, abortions and the emotional aspects of sexual intimacy?[9,10,11] The most common solution is to outsource this uncomfortable subject to the professionals.

Sex Education in Schools

What children learn about sex in formal sex-education classes obviously differs considerably depending on where your child goes to school in the world. Let's showcase a country that consistently leads the world in free-thinking and realistic damage-minimising strategies, Holland. In the Netherlands, it is often accepted as culturally appropriate to allow children of the same age to play doctors and nurses (even at school), so they can learn how to negotiate boundaries and consent from a young age and to limit sex-shaming.[12]

I agree that there is nothing unnatural about people being sexual with others in their same age group, even children exploring innocently with other children of either gender. According to the US Congress-founded National Child Traumatic Stress Network (NCTSN), this is considered natural and there is no evidence that children of the same age touching each

9. https://www.huffingtonpost.ca/entry/
    sex-education-pleasure_ca_5cd56c1ce4b07bc72977f516

10. https://www.salon.com/2018/09/13/
    take-the-shame-out-of-sex-ed-we-usually-start-with-the-risk-we-start-with-the-threat/

11. Breuner, Cora C., Gerri Mattson, and Committee on Psychosocial Aspects of Child and Family Health. 'Sexuality education for children and adolescents.' *Pediatrics* 138.2 (2016): e20161348.

12. https://www.thecut.com/2018/08/what-sex-education-is-like-in-the-netherlands.html

other leads to any sexual dysfunction.[13]

But even in very progressive countries such as Holland, there is still room for improvement. Worldwide researchers are finding a growing trend of sexual education failing, and the main reason given by students is because it is simply too dry, pretentious and clinical. The way most sex-education teachers talk about sex is nothing like the way the kids talk in the schoolyard. Obviously, it's important that children learn the correct names for things, but talking about sex like a doctor reading a medical journal seems to send a strong signal to kids that the adults would rather not be talking about this topic at all. *'Let's just get it over with, and with the least amount of emotion.'*[14,15]

For a long time, I have been offering to provide tantra sexual education to high-school students free of charge, but with the proviso that I would be allowed to speak graphically in street slang.[16] That offer has never been accepted. It seems the main reason is that parents get embarrassed, even listening to other adults graphically describing sex, let alone letting their *'darling-little-ones'* be exposed to that sort of foul language.

So, at the heart of the matter, it would seem the challenge is for parents to transcend their own sexual shame so that they don't pass on the imprint that sex is somehow wrong. There is evidence that adolescents can grow up to have a healthy sex life if they grew up in a household with a relaxed attitude towards sex.[17] Starting early seems to be the only way to help the child make the transition to the roller-coaster ride of teenage years. Without that, most adolescents go through a split state in which one part of them is still identified with the innocence of the child, while the other is subject to new and confusing hormone-driven wild horny, animal desires and their darker sexuality. Teenagers rarely have healthy role models to help them figure out how to reconcile those two parts of their psyche.

---

13. https://www.nctsn.org/sites/default/files/resources/sexual_development_and_behavior_in_children.pdf

14. https://www.latimes.com/local/lanow/la-me-sex-education-california-20190510-story.html

15. https://www.psychologytoday.com/us/blog/age-un-innocence/201801/should-parents-keep-sex-hush-hush

16. https://www.telegraph.co.uk/science/2017/11/20/sex-education-needs-graphic-teens-trying-taboo-practices-say/

17. https://www.telegraph.co.uk/family/schooling/graphic-sex-education-schools-isnt-just-good-idea-essential/

The old *'head-in-the-sand'* trick obviously doesn't work too well. Can you remember your youth? Didn't you feel that most of the adults were kind of dead, pretentious and fake when it came to the topic of sex? I certainly remember thinking that my parents had probably only ever had sex to procreate, plus a few extra times like wedding nights etc. If you've never seen your parents even kiss, learning that sex is a natural part of healthy adult interaction can be quite a shock.

Learning Boundaries

Learning boundaries can start even before a child can speak. In these days of heightened sensitivity to gaining consent before (and during) physical contact, it is increasingly important to teach children from the earliest of ages about bodily boundaries and how to say no. This can start even at the infant stage. You can nurture a child to develop good boundaries by laying down the *'groundwork for understanding bodily autonomy and consent'* by including them in decisions about what happens to them even on a most seemingly benign level of affection.[18] I routinely had to stop other people from unconsciously crossing boundaries by initiating unwanted affection to my daughter. People thought it was even rude if I did not allow a stranger on the bus to come and kiss my child on her head, or ruffle her hair. Although this is a well-intentioned and socially accepted behaviour, it sends a strong signal to the child that they can be touched without consent by someone they don't know, at any time. Even worse, it teaches them that refusing unwanted attention is somehow anti-social.

When you hold these boundaries, you may find that it hurts the feelings of a loving adult who wants to express their affection for your child, but isn't it better for an adult to have a moment of awkwardness, than to teach your child they have to allow access to their bodies just because someone else wants it?[19]

Photo credit: *Mores345* (https://pixabay.com/users/mores345-3611991/), https://pixabay.com/photos/holding-hands-love-relationship-1772035/

---

18. https://www.parents.com/parenting/better-parenting/advice/how-to-teach-your-child-about-consent-from-birth/

19. https://www.washingtonpost.com/lifestyle/2018/10/16/ways-parents-can-help-kids-understand-consent-prevent-sexual-assault/

47

I KNOW HOW TO PARTY

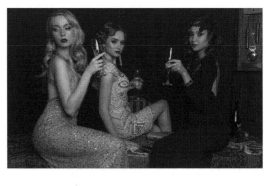

Raising the Party Bar

Many people think that with enough money you can have an amazing party.[1] However, this is not necessarily the case. I've been in the privileged position to have taught and hung out with people in the movie industry in Hollywood. (No, I won't drop any names. I think privacy is highly underrated).

Films and television paint an artificially cool picture of Hollywood parties being wild and free. The slightly disappointing reality was that it doesn't matter where I travelled in the world, or how much money people throw at a party, they rarely lived up to the hyped-up expectations, and weren't nearly as fun as our sexual de-conditioning workshop parties at The New Tantra. Disappointingly so...

The Dionysian is no picnic. —Camille Paglia

There's a couple of reasons for this. Most people's idea of an incredible night would probably involve great sex at some stage of the evening, but amazing sex prowess is not something that can be simply bought. Even if you get invited to the jet-set sex parties, they all seem to suffer the same problem... everybody who is non-Tantric will lose energy after the regular

---

1. https://www.businessinsider.com/inside-snctm-the-mysterious-los-angeles-sex-club-2018-1#while-no-new-names-are-yet-to-be-leaked-snctm-has-said-they-are-taking-measures-to-protect-the-privacy-of-members-10

orgasm.[2,3,4] Combine that with the usual ego contraction that makes people take themselves too seriously and you might start to get a more realistic picture that most parties are just... meh.[5,6]

The other reason why parties don't often live up to their expectations is that people simply aren't educated in modern tantric sex practices that they can apply to Western life in the 21st century. If people could learn some new skills while building up their energy, become better lovers and have one of the best nights of their lives at a mind-blowing party, that would be a win-win situation for everybody.

The reason I used the phrase *'disappointingly so'* earlier is that it doesn't really work for me to go to cool TNT parties myself. The problem is when the founder walks in, the room often becomes rather self-conscious and strained. It's not a relaxing scenario for any of us, so I spend most of the time alone or with a few of my close female friends. Therefore, I'm very happy to attend other cool parties, but the more exposure I get to the so-called exclusive jet-set festivities, the more potential I see in taking them to the next level.

Experienced facilitators can create deep tantric spaces. If you are interested, there is some more information on this footnote.[7]

Photo credit: *Anastasia Gepp* (https://pixabay.com/users/nastya_gepp-3773230/), https://pixabay.com/photos/three-women-fashion-hair-glamour-3075752/

---

2. https://www.insider.com/why-sex-makes-you-sleepy-2018-3

3. https://www.livescience.com/32445-why-do-guys-get-sleepy-after-sex.html

4. https://www.bustle.com/p/why-some-people-feel-tired-after-sex-8590759

5. https://www.cosmopolitan.com/uk/love-sex/sex/a9558003/killing-kittens-sex-party-elite-london/

6. https://www.latimes.com/entertainment-arts/story/2020-02-04/hollywood-oscar-party-crasher-adrian-maher-remembers

7. The *'TNT Tantric Party Starters'* program, which works something like this. You pay a donation and fly a bunch of 10 to 20 highly-trained (and hot) TNT Tantric practitioners (of varying ages and genders) to turn up to your party. We start with an hour or so of theory and Tantric education and then we do instructional demonstrations to get the party really started. I've been instructing at some of the most famous upmarket libertine society parties and it interests me to see how much people are willing to learn and experiment if there is a higher purpose for learning new skills. The larger the donation and the more fun the party is for our group, the longer we stay. I am told having a few really open people to lead the tantric way makes a much bigger talking point than the label of French champagne was being served! For more information, send a message through the contact form on www.50misconceptionsofsex.com.

48

MEN CHASE WOMEN

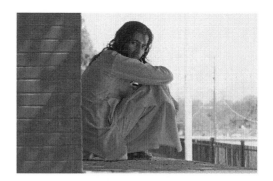

Usually, But Not Always

I'm a profoundly lazy sex... er... machine? More like a rusty, old Lancia Delta Integrale Evolution from the early '90s, to be fair. Sure, that rally car went like *'stink'* in it's prime, but these days it might cost you a lot more than what it's worth if you took it to the redline. I don't really know how I got so lazy about sex. Maybe it's an occupational hazard? Perhaps, a side-effect of practising various forms of tantra since 2001 is that it all gets a bit ho-hum. I haven't heard of many gynaecologists getting tired of pussies after looking at them all day long, but somehow, something akin to this happened to me. I will shed some light on this topic because if you practise the principles of this book, the same may very well happen to you, guys. So, it's good to be prepared, as I see it happen quite a lot with tantric practitioners who achieve a certain level of sexual prowess.

My colleagues used to joke at how they could predict my usual rapid *'exit stage right'* as soon as the clothes would come off in The New Tantra Level 2 Advanced sex workshops. This was followed by me, squeamishly handing over the mic to my co-facilitators in my dash for a little Netflix series-binging. It would seem that *everything* that is over-supplied loses its appeal if it is done in both quantity and quality.

It wasn't always like that. Many years ago, I used to love being the man and having sex with women, but I think in the last 10 years I can only remember trying to pick up one woman, (and that was a dare from a colleague to see if I could still get my game on). That's the main reason why, on the rare occasions that I do have sex, it is with men (or women that are willing to do the hard masculine *'topping'* work).

Having been a tantra workshop facilitator puts one in a rare position that few people seem able to relate to. Before tantra, men chased women. It seems totally ingrained in humans that this is the way for everyone but the super-rich, like movie actors and rock stars (a difficult crowd to join). But on a more ordinary level, once you master tantra, women chase the tantrically-accomplished men. You can't believe the trouble I have got in the past for *not* having sex with some women. Women (unlike men), don't seem to have such a thick hide when it comes to sexual rejection.

Being someone who is attracted to dominant people means the whole dynamic of having people looking up to you as the alpha is inherently un-appealing. Self-imposing a 3-year *'no-go-zone'* if a woman came to one of my workshops was one way to address the issue. I used to say to female participants *'you wouldn't even give me the time of day if I tried to pick you up in a club'*. It is only in a workshop environment that the facilitator has an artificial alpha desirability due to their position. Taking advantage of that is kind of sleazy. Same reason why U2 doesn't allow groupies backstage.[1]

Don't get me wrong, I love the look and beauty of women over a man's any day, but what I also see is a huge amount of work and a lot of investment in time and energy to help a non-tantric woman become fully-functional in the tantric sense. De-armouring their bodies to get them vulnerable, then activating their spine sexually, then de-armouring their vagina, g-spot, cervix and finally spending a huge amount of energy doing tonnes of push-ups for hours on end. I get tired just thinking about it.[2]

So, being sexual with a man is totally different. I get to lie on the mat-tress and receive pleasure without having to do much physical work or direct the show. It's a much better deal, in my eyes! Being attracted to the feminine form equates to the man helping me get horny on my *own* feminine side by making me feel the desired female.

Anyway, to give you a little deeper taste into my world and what it was like to be in a tantric relationship (as a man) with a woman (and the amount of energy it takes), I cast my memories way back to a past relationship.

---

1. https://www.nytimes.com/1997/08/31/theater/backstage-a-whole-other-show-goes-on.html

2. https://www.thedailymeal.com/healthy-eating/7-exercises-improve-your-sexual-stamina-slideshow/slide-6

50 MISCONCEPTIONS OF SEX

Reader discretion is advised...

> I'm delighted that my lover has arrived. She is animated and profoundly brilliant. We spend hours in deep spiritual conversation, sometimes agreeing and sometimes pushing each other to reassess our beliefs. I love this woman, but it is not a love shaped by duty or social pressure. I don't stay with her out of habit or fear of loneliness. Instead, our love is driven by an authentic spiritual, mental and physical connection. We grow more quickly because we choose to walk this spiritual path together.

> Although she is beautiful and successful in her career, her spiritual longing keeps her humble. I enjoy her company and am content with her companionship and conversation, but I am also paying attention to her body language. I like to anticipate her needs so she doesn't have to tell me where she would like to be taken. Right now, I'm noticing that her energy seems a bit low and she appears a little restless. I notice that she has been touching me casually. I know her well enough that sitting and talking is not going to be enough for her much longer. She seems to shorten her sentences, perhaps signalling a desire for a more physical interaction.

> She's wearing a form-fitting business dress with a deep slit, and I can just see the top of her stocking peeking out. I know there is more than a clever mind, she can be alive with sexual energy. I am mindful about how I start our sexual play. I have spent time studying the type of language that turns most women on, and I learned from experience what works specifically for her, through trial and error. I have to push past my nice-guy conditioning. If I were to stick with what's politically-correct and socially-acceptable, I might say something like, 'Would you like to join me in the bedroom?' But that would leave her panties crispy dry and perhaps elicit a concealed yawn. I would need to do better.

Although many women who have had their hearts broken think that they only ever want to be treated and spoken gently by men, it's been my experience that the best in a women will quickly find *'gentle mode'* boring and un-arousing if done all the time.[3] That is why there are sayings like *'nice guys finish last'* and *'women want bad boys.'*[4] The truth is a little more complicated, of course... Within the boundaries of a relationship in which

3. https://www.psychologytoday.com/us/blog/head-games/201310/why-do-women-fall-bad-boys
4. https://www.psychologytoday.com/us/blog/the-attraction-doctor/201501/nice-guys-or-bad-boys-what-do-women-want

trust and respect have been established, women often want the guys to direct and take the initiative.

Timing is everything, so I tune into what her feminine side yearns to hear, right now. Although I know that this sentence might rightfully garner me a slap in the face in a bar, I test whether this is the right moment to grow a pair and man up.

'I'm afraid I'm having some difficulty concentrating on what you're saying. You look way too hot sitting there in that dress. Maybe it's time I moved you somewhere more interesting and fucked you a little bit? Hmmm?'

'Yes, please!' She responds. Her voice raises in pitch as more energy suddenly enters her body. She suddenly sounds more like an eighteen-year-old girl than a businesswoman... while I work my poker face and attempt to conceal my relief that my intuition was right. She's been in her head all day, and now she's ready to be in her body more, but she needs a little masculine help and direction to make that transition.

She turns to walk ahead of me, but I grab her by the waist and spin her around. 'Just where do you think you're going, you little vixen? Are you decid-ing where you're gonna be taken to? Is that how this is going to work?' I smirk at her with one raised eyebrow. She gives me a sheepish look. She knows this is all part of the game, so it's fun for her to act a little small and be reminded that she can take a temporary break from being in charge of her actions.

In our daily life, she is independent and has a lot of responsibilities. She doesn't need to be taken care of, and she doesn't need me to solve her prob-lems. She is more capable than me at so many things... and can be quite dominant as well... so we both know that she is surrendering to me right now because she is longing to put down her masculine side and soften in the freedom of not having to make any decisions for a while, and simply follow me and show me with her body if it is working.

The more structure I provide, the more she can surrender. Still holding her by the waist, I pull her close to me and press her body to mine. With my arms tightly wrapped around her, my body becomes her temporary exoskeleton. She can fully relax her body with me as support. My cock is sensitive to her surrender and is quick to react... especially as I have not ejaculated in a few months. The warmth and softness of her athletic body make me hard right away. She takes a deep breath and relaxes her muscles; the boundary where our bodies touch starts to melt away. With every intentional breath, I can feel her following me and becoming synchronised with the rhythm of my chest.

At this moment, I can feel an aching constriction, as the right side of my chest opens energetically into her chest. I'm not a very woo-woo kind of a person, but at this moment, it feels as though her heart is opening up in response to the demand of my love. Logically, I know that this is probably just my imagination, but maybe all our perception of reality is just a projection of some sort of greater mind... so why not go with it, especially since she seems to respond in perfect synchronicity to my internal feeling of how open my heart is, moment-to-moment... and where I direct my attention inside her. She says she already feels me inside her and she can predict with uncanny accuracy which part of her body I am focusing on, internally.

I use my hands to help her surrender deeper... not just to me... but to everything around us, to the Universe, to Spirit, to Love, whatever you want to call it. The intention is to connect to something greater than ourselves.[5]

I move my hands to her spine, and it starts to undulate without her conscious control. She had her spine sexually activated years ago, and that movement seems to let her go into a sort of light trance state. Each breath she draws in is slow and long. Her body is relaxed, alert and alive.

I walk her back into the bedroom. Her eyes are now on mine, and she can feel that I know what her body longs for, deeper than her own mind can access. There is no need for her to adhere to social conventions. She doesn't need to play the 'hard-to-get' game, withholding sex from the greedy man...[6] Instead, we are equals, agreeing to play certain roles together. She showed her decision to let go when I first challenged her as she tried to lead the way to the bedroom.

'Clothes off... leave the lingerie on, lie on the bed, it's time to play!' I instantly check for consent... or if I have overstepped my permission field. Her smile and bedroom eyes leave no doubt that I haven't.

Even though I know that I am doing this for her benefit, there is still a part of my mind that finds these kinds of words utterly cringeworthy. They remind me all too well of the macho Australian jerks that I detested so much, growing up. It took much practise and instruction from my teachers (and confirmation from many women), to learn that most female people

---

5. Maybe that's what they refer to as the *'oceanic feeling'* in psychology and sociology. https://www.encyclopedia.com/psychology/dictionaries-thesauruses-pictures-and-press-releases/oceanic-feeling

6. https://www.psychologytoday.com/us/blog/the-attraction-doctor/201606/how-and-why-play-hard-get

get bored with *'too sweet'* and *'too nice'*... and through practice, I learned how to address that longing. It certainly wasn't intuitive for me... to say the least![7]

> *I take my clothes off and lie down on top of her. I'm intentionally making her wait longer than she might expect, as a way to increase her desire. Foreplay, at this point, would be too much for her. My direction, words and power exchange has been more than enough preparation... for now, at least... We might circle back to foreplay after the intermission break for the proverbial sexual snacks, so to speak... but right now, she needs more substance.*

To be continued...

Photo credit: *Devanath* (https://pixabay.com/users/devanath-1785462/), https://pixabay.com/photos/man-wall-portrait-india-young-1103133/

---

7. https://www.psychologytoday.com/us/blog/meet-catch-and-keep/201405/do-nice-guys-really-finish-last

49

SEX IS FUN
For Whom?

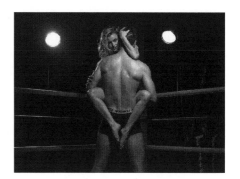

Because sex is a hobby for most people, it firmly lies in the realm of pleasure and fun... but sex can also be a valuable gift of shared yoga that can ripple into many other areas of life but can also be a lot of work for the active partner.[1]

> Gently, but with clear direction and intent, I slowly enter her pussy. She gasps... the right mix of a pleasurable groan and an edgy, surprised involuntary inhaled 'Oh!' I hold it there without movement to give her time to get used to the fullness of flesh and masculine demand. No friction at this point. We are both sensitive enough to feel each other without having to do the mutual genital massage thang.

> I look deeply into her eyes, past the familiar face that I usually see, to some aspect of her more universal and ever-refreshed self. She is less self-reflective and thus more confident in her body, eyes and facial expression. The more she positively responds, the more I know she is with me and can relax into where this train seems to be taking us, which I certainly don't know (although it may seem to her that I do). Not knowing when or what is going to happen next gives her the pleasure of constant surprise.

Incidentally... in my 20's, I used to spend a lot of time on clitoral stimulation to give the woman a few quick orgasms. I had some good techniques down there and was naive enough to think this made me a good lover. It was years later when I slept with the partner of another tantra practitioner that I learned from some honest and rather painful feedback that my techniques made for boring sex. My well-rehearsed routine was smashed in one night, and I had nothing to fall back on. It took many years to learn

---

1. https://www.huffpost.com/entry/healing-sex_b_2666015

new theory and practices before I felt confident enough to trust my own sexual intuition.

Sex has a way to shatter rigid identities and rigid ways of being and thinking. I found out that addressing these issues had repercussions far beyond my sex life.

> She can feel the horny energy building up in my penis. I feel the sensation that most men briefly know when they are around 95% of the way and rushing to climax. But I slow down to keep the heat simmering. Somehow, she can feel what she refers to as a 'buzzing with sexual electricity' or 'the humming cock'... A cock that needs no friction to be felt.

Incidentally, I first learned about the 'humming cock' when a past lover was describing our sexual encounters to a friend. I had no idea the woman could actually feel the same sensation I was feeling without any movement. My point is that there seems to be a different level of sensitivity in tantra that can make even boring looking sex really interesting.

> She's getting a little too carried away now. She starts to writhe beneath me, angling her hips and wiggling her butt. I grab her hips and say 'No, too much' as I slide half out. I just received an internal danger signal that took me a long time to learn to register... a dangerous sudden subtle energy flash going up the front of my body. If she had continued, I would have gone over the edge.

Even though the physical refractory period might allow for a second attempt, my penis would be much less sensitive and not able to produce the frictionless-sex energy.[2] I wouldn't feel shit if I wasn't moving and, as I learned the hard way, neither would she. More on this in a minute.

> I stay present and try to only think about what is actually happening in the room... while at the same time not over-focusing on the non-cumming thing... kind of like that pink elephant analogy. I slide inside again ever so slowly, this time playing at the opening, back and forth with some super slippery action, just to tease her... before I slide fully into her when she doesn't expect it. Her surprised moan of satisfaction is the repayment for not teasing her too long.

I'm glad that she is committed to this tantric practice. She has long transcended the addiction to cumming via the clitoral pudendal nerve and instead prefers the deeper tantric orgasms. Long ago, she lost the superficial, feminine need to show she was desirable and hot by making men cum.

---

2. https://www.healthline.com/health/healthy-sex/refractory-period

The problem, though, is that she has lost all interest in having sex with non-tantric men... although she is certainly free to do so. I have little fear that she will stray too far from tantric pleasures. I would love more men to *'share the workload'* as well as allow others to enjoy this amazing woman, but besides one other tantric lover, she's not so interested in non-tantric men and would rather play sexually with women instead.

Because she doesn't let men dump their stress in her body or indulge in the clitoral spasm orgasms, her vagina and cervix are soft and pulse with an energy that we found out (the hard way), is too much horniness for non-tantric guys.

I further allow the intelligence of our bodies to take over. I've set something in motion, and now I just need to mentally get out of the way and see where this is going to go. Instead of deciding to hold her 'like this' and squeeze her 'like that', I surrender to an intuitive greater knowing and flow of energy that allows our bodies to respond, unhindered by our conscious minds.

There is more movement and friction now, but not in any predictable way. She is getting lost in her sensations as she should be, but I cannot be un-present for even a moment. I don't have the luxury of self-indulgently losing myself in sensations. It's like meditating; two people entering into a flow state at the same time.

I spontaneously begin dirty-talking to her and testing what makes her body respond. Does she start breathing more heavily and pressing her body more fully when I tell her to confess her desire? Let's test it and see...

'You seem to be enjoying some tantric cock there?'

'Yes! Oh, yes!'

OK. Let's take it a little further and see if that's where she wants to go. Honestly, a part of me would be really content to stay where we are... but there is no arguing with the flow of a woman's body.

'Would you like me to put it where only the really naughty girls like it? Deep in your pussy, up against your cervix?' I press my cock hard against the opening to her womb.

'Is that where you like it?'

'Oh yes!.... like that...there, there.... yes... more... please!'

'Ah... so you are one of those dirty little girls that like to be really well fucked!'

'Ya... Ya!'

Instantly, her cervix feels electric.

I have to be careful in these early moments. Any one of those electric sparks could catch me by surprise and ignite a fire in me that moves quickly and dangerously up the front of my body, causing me to ejaculate uncontrollably... with little warning. How embarrassing would that be! TILT, GAME OVER!

As I mentioned earlier, I could possibly rally for a second round, but the sexual energy in our bodies would only be a fraction of what it is after months of saving and circulating that energy. A failure or mistake at this point would also reinforce her bodily belief that her sexual energy is too much for me. This would make it so much more difficult for her to trust that she can fully let go and not hold back in fear of overwhelming me. This will prevent her from experiencing the womb orgasm because she will hold back her deepest surrender and stop right before she *energetically* opens her cervix and allows the shockwaves from the pounded cervix to vibrate her womb into orgasmic submission.

Furthermore, a second rallying, (something I call *'getting back in the saddle'*) is a dangerous move, as the instant-gratification, clenching reflex has just been recently activated and is reinforced in me. The old habit of squeezing for a few seconds to intensify the release pleasure never really dies... It just gets more distant, the further from the last time you did it.

I focus my intention back towards my ass and spine, and the energy weirdly seems to follow. This seems to spread the energy throughout my body so that it doesn't build up too much in my base and overload my system.

I can't do a lot of friction at this early stage, as that would create too much stimulation for me, so I stay deep inside and bump against her cervix with only short withdrawing strokes. She seems to be going crazy and responds more, the harder I bump. On a particularly deep thrust against her cervix, I notice her breathing momentarily stops and I notice a brief wince cross her face.

'Is there any pain there?'

'Yes, a little... right there'

'Remember, babe... you have to tell me that. I don't read minds, and I don't want to hurt you.'

Now, she drops the habit of resisting and tensing against the pain and allows me to hear her vulnerability... 'ouch, ooooooh, awwww, fuck, mamma

mamma... right there! Shit!...aghhh!' Her sounds and words are much easier instructions to understand. Somehow, expressing the sounds of pain help her be vulnerable and let go of that deepest pain through externalising it in vocal expression.

I press and hold hard against her cervix, but hearing her pain is making my dick go limp. This is the part of the session I dislike the most. I need to move a little to create some friction to maintain my erection. A few slippery strokes and it thankfully returns. The de-armouring continues.

'Push that pain out into my cock. It doesn't harm my cock. Don't leave any of that shit in there. Push it out a little more.'

After a minute or so, the sounds cease, and pain seems to have gone. Now she says it feels good. I test by pressing even harder and double-checking verbally.

'Even like that?' I am now pressing as hard as I can, to the point where my dick would bruise if I pressed any harder. I test the cervix with an even harder and deeper thrust.

'OK?'

She nods affirmatively with her body responding with an even stronger 'yes' to that question. Her shyness (learned from an embarrassed mother telling her not to be a slut), dissolves in overwhelming pleasure beyond any previous sexual conditioning.

'Oh yes! Fuck me, fuck me! like that! Ohhhh, God. Yes!'

I am always a little scared that I will hurt her, and I need some extra verbal encouragement that I'm not abusing her.

I move on to the next stage, which I call 'mashing the potatoes'. The cervix can be felt like a nose, distinctly at the back of the vagina. My cock instinctively targets that point with deep rhythmic thrusts, and our external flesh is making loud slapping sounds. Inside, the cervix is physically starting to dilate by about 1/2 cm, with extreme horniness... and that opening is enough to act as a gateway to allow those shockwaves to shake the womb.

I move her into the most vulnerable position. I place both her legs over my shoulders. This exposes her cervix much more. I press and thrust with caution as I know through experience that women will always pick up stress throughout the day and store it here... and there always seems to be a little bit of tension remaining right in the centre.

'Ouch, yes, right there!'

'Good. You tell me...'

Within 1 or 2 minutes of pressing and holding, we're mashing the potatoes on max setting. This time, she seems even wilder and more demanding. It's just as well that I've been going to the gym lately!

Within only a few minutes, she seems to be slipping into 'super slut mode'.

It's no shock to me. Here's something most people fail to imagine. At this deepest level of sexual yoga, there is **zero** variation. It seems that all women have the same way of functioning when it comes to the internal sexual yoga of the cervix and womb orgasm.[3] You learn one and you learn them all.

I know where this is going. So I continue to mash that potato with all I've got...

'Fuck me, fuck me, harder, harder!'

Sweat is raining down on her face. Now I need to resort to my secret weapon. It's something that feels like controlled anger... but as a gift... for her sake.

Getting her to fully own her dark side, I hear myself constantly talking in ways that sound to my ears as borderline abusive... but her response says otherwise.

'You want me to fuck you right there...? Like that...? Do you?'

'Yes please... just like that... like that! Please don't stop! Don't stop, please don't stop!'

'You want me to fuck you like a dirty little slut then? Like this?'

'Yes, oh fuck yes, I'm a dirty girl! I like that, I like that!'

At this point, she has lost all awareness of the outside world. I am getting worried about my neighbours.

One of our gigolos in Holland had the police turn up on his doorstep and almost break down the door.[4] A concerned neighbour thought that some poor girl was being raped. Luckily, the client came out with a sheet wrapped around her and explained in a matter-of-fact mindless state that she was being taught tantra and was having *'the best sex of her life!'* The police laughed and suggested maybe screaming into a pillow for the neigh-

---

3. https://www.tandfonline.com/doi/abs/10.1080/10532528.2005.10559829

4. https://www.thenewtantra.com/private-sessions

bours' sake. Then, they wrote down our website address and one of them even came later to an intro talk.[5] Gotta love Holland!

Anyway, back to the present.

She is now entering womb orgasm.

A lot of tantric women mistakenly think they have had a womb orgasm. It is not exactly subtle or difficult to detect when one actually does occur.

Her vagina starts sucking in huge amounts of air and forcefully expelling it with every vaginal contraction. I alternate between not being able to feel any friction as her vagina has turned into a balloon... and contracting so hard that I can hardly enter her vagina as it is involuntarily clenched like a fist. If I need to push much harder and slip, it will feel as if I would snap my dick in half. (That's a real thing, you know...),[6] but ramming it through her tightness sends her over the top into la-la-land. Fart, fart, fart, fart! Can't... stop... now.... the show, must... go... on...

More fuck talk and I have to grab a towel to put under her ass as she is totally losing control and continuously softly squirting on my cock whenever I command her to. She doesn't seem to know who or what she is anymore. She has very little mind left, to the point where the room and our bodies are glowing in an effervescent green, and it is virtually impossible to think or even form memories.

Incidentally, on the first meeting, our tantric cock master Maya, a hot Brazilian transsexual, could not remember our 2-hour mindless tantric sex initiation the night before the following day. And she was a very experienced girl to say the least. Anyway, I digress...

At this point, I can also make her orgasm without any movement. I simply place the most horny energy in my cock and let that horny energy expand into her vagina or cervix and tell her body what to feel.

As soon as I notice any predictable routine starting, I unexpectedly flip her into a different position. I take her from behind, then on her side. Sometimes hard, sometimes soft... sometimes back to no movement. I simply don't interfere. I call it extreme 'yogic laziness' to not make an effort to stop what The Greater whispers through the intuition of what to do next.

I feel like I've run a half-marathon. So we change gears. Softly, gently caress-

---

5. https://www.thenewtantra.com/
6. https://en.wikipedia.org/wiki/Penile_fracture

ing her while admiring her body. I'm gazing deeply into her eyes, tears well up in the meeting of something that is the same in both of us, recognising each other in the opposite of otherness. This is actually my favourite part. Not having to do anything and just experiencing the energetic warmth of our hearts ripping open. My consciousness expands as far out as I can comprehend, I feel as if I am the container in which everything appears. And there she is... meeting me there and ripping my heart so far open until it physically hurts in my chest.

Her face looks more beautiful than I have ever seen before. The sensation is as if I'm seeing her for the first time. And now this adult woman looks like a glowing young girl. I can't find any resistance to fall into her unending transfiguration into something that resembles my idea of the divine goddess in human form.

Quantity and variety of sex have been rapidly replaced by an appreciation for quality and depth. This is a depth that I can only find with a person I am committed to loving.

Reading this first-hand account hopefully graphically relays the message that sex is not always about hedonistic pleasure but can also be a spiritually transcendent experience without the use of drugs and a deep and life changing service to another.[7] Many meditations in Hinduism and Buddhism involve visualising deities (yiddam practice),[8] but rather than sitting on a pillow, one can reach these meditative states using transcendent sex.

Photo credit: *Lonzu* (https://pixabay.com/users/longzu-6105256/), https://pixabay.com/photos/love-woman-sexy-brave-2784238/

7. https://www.psychologytoday.com/us/blog/love-without-limits/201408/why-sex-is-sacred

8. https://vividness.live/2017/02/09/yidams-a-godless-approach-naturally/

50

SEX ISN'T ALTRUISTIC

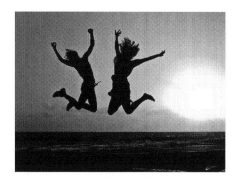

For the Greater Good

Writing this book was a labour of love. The main thing that kept me going through my multiple phases of resistance was thinking that it might help others, and especially future generations. I want people to have access to this information so they can test and see if it works for them. Maybe it will even create a slightly better world, as so many problems seem to have deep sexual roots. Screwed-up adults, who grew out of screwed-up families that harboured screwed-up sexual issues, that end up running screwed up societies. We have probably all witnessed first-hand the damage that sex can do to a family, business and country.

I would have loved to grow up in a more relaxed world without so much shame, repression and sexual-dysfunction. So, if only a few people ever read this book, at least I know I did my best to try to create a modern form of tantra that brings together wisdom old and new, from ancient meditation traditions, to philosophy and modern science. So where to start?

Communication

The key to solving most problems starts with communication, but when it comes to talking about sex, there is often an invisible *'cone of silence'* in the form of shame. Thus, lack of communication means that many wounds will go unhealed, and many sexual problems will silently pass from one generation to the next. It is, therefore, likely that if we are going to have any chance to truly help our children live healthy, natural sex-lives, we have to achieve that for ourselves first.

If there is anything that we wish to change in the child, we should first examine

it and see whether it is not something that could better be changed in ourselves.
—Carl Gustav Jung (1875-1961), Swiss psychiatrist and psychoanalyst

Prevention is Better than Cure

As for the Nature Vs Nurture debate, I believe we are born at our purest potential, so it is mainly an unhealthy social environment and upbringing that distorts us. By pure, I mean we are born with the potential for physical, spiritual, mental and emotional wellbeing... but when learnt emotions like guilt and shame are inflicted on our children, they reduce the likelihood of them growing into healthy, happy and functional adults. Undoing the damage that has been done to them through therapy, or simply living a deeply-questioned life is painstaking and difficult, to say the least. It would seem easier to avoid damaging the child in the first place.

It is an unfortunate fact that most people spend more planning, preparing and getting approval to build a garage than they do to have a child. If you wish to change that situation and do some basic preparations, here are some practical tips for conceiving and raising a child with as little damage as possible:

Shameless Sex

First step in this preparation would be practising tantra and, thus, getting away from the more guilt-laden orgasms. Naturally, the shameless enjoyment of sex should help create a healthier imprint for your upcoming child by the way you live. How might your child develop differently from the way we did if you allow them to grow up in a sexually-relaxed home environment? A place where sex is seen as a natural part of life and not something that makes everyone around the dinner table squirm? From the first questions of *'Where do babies come from?'* there can be shameless matter-of-fact discussions if the parents are sexually de-conditioned themselves.

Even before cognisant capacities have developed, babies are constantly learning. When a child touches their genitalia, can the parents be relaxed enough to allow them to innocently explore their bodies? Or do they embarrassingly move their hands away with a tap and a *'no'*? Sure, you can later gently educate them about appropriate behaviour and the difference between public and private settings to avoid other people's discomfort, but my advice is to make it clear that there is absolutely nothing wrong with self-exploration and self-pleasuring in private. The child at that age only wants to please and be loved, so a strong signal that it is wrong to feel sexual self-pleasure can have a strong guilt-producing, sub-conscious influence for the rest of their life.

Planned Birth

Instead of being born a mistake (40% of pregnancies are unintended),[1] wouldn't it be preferable to know parents planned the night of conception intentionally, creating an atmosphere of beauty and love that illustrated their love of each other and their reverence for their future, desired child? The Tibetans seem to believe that the setting, intention and love between the parents are factors in determining the level of consciousness of the child.[2] No way to prove that one scientifically, but I guess it can't hurt.

Orgasmic Birth

What better way to come into the world than with your mother in a state of orgasmic uterine euphoria rather than intense pain or cloudy anaesthetics? As we discussed in chapter 27 There is a whole movement now called *'Orgasmic Birth'*.[3] Mothers-to-be will benefit greatly if they are able to orgasm on the cervix and womb before becoming pregnant. If a woman is able to experience these types of orgasms during tantric sex, she will more than likely have a pain-free, orgasmic birth. Google it yourself, if you don't believe it, and see what's possible.[4]

If you are already pregnant, there are professionally trained midwives that have included the tantric knowledge of cervix de-armouring into their existing professional practices. Through early-term cervical massage, they can soften the cervix to allow for a greatly-reduced and even pain-free orgasmic birth.

1. https://www.ncbi.nlm.nih.gov/pmc/articles/PMC4727534/

2. Brown, A.M., Farwell, E., and Nyerongsha, D. (2008) *The Tibetan Art of Parenting—From Before Conception through Early Childhood*. Wisdom Publications, Boston USA 2008. ISBN 0-86171-579-9.

3. https://www.orgasmicbirth.com/about/what-is-orgasmic-birth/

4. https://www.glamour.com/story/whats-it-actually-like-to-have-an-orgasmic-birth

Home Birth?

Although parents need to decide for themselves what they think is best for their upcoming birthing situation, one of the most natural and comfortable ways to give birth is at home and preferably in water. Of course, it's important to have a fully-trained and equipped midwife who knows how to handle emergencies like haemorrhaging, in case something goes wrong. Having a plan B is sensible in any situation, and rarely more than in birth situations. How close is your home to medical services in case something does go wrong? Do you have a written birth plan that covers as many logistics and possible scenarios?

Statistically, it is as safe to have a planned birth at home as it is in a hospital if you have a normally-presenting baby and no high-risk factors:

A large international study led by McMaster University shows that low-risk pregnant women who intend to give birth at home have no increased chance of the baby's perinatal or neonatal death compared to other low-risk women who intend to give birth in a hospital.[5]

Planned home births generally result in a high level of satisfaction with the birth experience,[6,7] plus they give the women more control over the childbirth process. With more decision-making power over medical interventions and more freedom to birth on their body's schedule (rather than on the doctors' schedules).[8] Increased autonomy and emotional support during home births can create a more natural and relaxed atmosphere for giving birth.[9,10]

On the contrary, some women will be able to relax more in a hospital setting, knowing that if anything does go wrong help is close at hand,

---

5. https://www.sciencedaily.com/releases/2019/08/190807190818.htm

6. https://www.ncbi.nlm.nih.gov/pmc/articles/PMC2742137/

7. Zielinski R, Ackerson K, Kane Low L. Planned home birth: benefits, risks, and opportunities. *Int J Womens Health.* 2015;7:361–377. Published 2015 Apr 8. doi:10.2147/IJWH.S55561

8. Armstrong EM. Home birth matters-for all women. *J Perinat Educ.* 2010;19(1):8–11. doi:10.1624/105812410X482329

9. https://www.npr.org/sections/health-shots/2019/03/11/700829719/home-birth-can-be-appealing-but-how-safe-is-it

10. https://parenting.nytimes.com/pregnancy/home-birth

and they won't face the resistance of bucking current societal conventions. Each to their own.

Attachment Parenting

Attachment parenting or *'sensitive and responsive parenting'*, can have a huge impact on how the child acts later in life.[11] There is a lot of information on this subject, but in a nutshell, it is about raising children who feel secure by responding to their needs in a timely and age-appropriate manner.[12] One important aspect of this is physical skin-on-skin contact from birth between the child and at least one parent at all times, for at least the first 6 months. This reinforces in the infant's somatic nervous system that they are safe and loved.[13,14] It's the opposite of wrapping your baby in clothes, giving it a bottle and leaving it to cry itself into submission in its crib, in a separate room!

Some of the methods of attachment parenting, like co-sleeping, slings (instead of prams) and breastfeeding until at least two years of age as recommended by the W.H.O.,[15] are a huge commitment and take a massive amount of work (especially for the mother!) The upside is that this early investment in energy is usually paid back multiple times as the child matures. Taking the time to understand and empathetically respond to an infant's needs seems to result in a child that is far more emotionally-mature and independent. Frustrating behaviours like endless attention-seeking and panic when the parent is out of sight can

11. https://www.parentingscience.com/attachment-parenting.html

12. https://www.psychologytoday.com/us/blog/fulfillment-any-age/201307/the-4-principles-attachment-parenting-and-why-they-work?destination=node/128865

13. Crenshaw JT. Healthy Birth Practice #6: Keep Mother and Baby Together—It's Best for Mother, Baby, and Breastfeeding. *J Perinat Educ.* 2014;23(4):211–217. doi:10.1891/1058-1243.23.4.211

14. Er-Mei Chen, Meei-Ling Gau, Chieh-Yu Liu, and Tzu-Ying Lee, 'Effects of Father-Neonate Skin-to-Skin Contact on Attachment: A Randomized Controlled Trial,' *Nursing Research and Practice*, vol. 2017, Article ID 8612024, 8 pages, 2017. https://doi.org/10.1155/2017/8612024.

15. https://www.who.int/news-room/fact-sheets/detail/infant-and-young-child-feeding

greatly diminish with an emotionally-secure child.[16,17]

Authoritative Parenting

Hand-in-hand with attachment parenting is *authoritative* parenting. This method focuses on high responsiveness to the child's needs while communicating and treating the child with the same rights and respect as an adult.[18] When parents engage in authoritative parenting, they nurture their children's ability to handle frustration. They also better understand their child's perspective and thus can provide an age-appropriate explanation to help the child understand *why* certain boundaries have been set.[19]

This should not be confused with *authoritarian* parenting, with high expectations of the child but with low responsiveness to the child's needs.[20] Rules are enforced with shame, yelling, and excessively harsh punishment and the child's perspective is not considered. A classic old-time lazy authoritarian suppression technique is *'because I say so'*. It's a hallmark of tired and frustrated parents that don't have the energy to explain the reason why of their rules. Now, imagine for a moment saying that to an adult! The damage done through lack of respect can set a bad foundation for the child's relationship with any authority figure in the future. Children raised by authoritarian parents are also generally less self-reliant, more socially-awkward and more likely to be bullies.

Bully-Free Education

The trauma from peer-bullying has been shown to affect people into their adult years, and it should *not* (as has traditionally been) be viewed a normal part of growing up or a *'rite of passage'* into adulthood, according to Dieter Wolke and Suzet Tanya Lereya, from the Department of

---

16. Mary D. Salter Ainsworth, and Silvia M. Bell. 'Attachment, Exploration, and Separation: Illustrated by the Behavior of One-Year-Olds in a Strange Situation.' *Child Development*, vol. 41, no. 1, 1970, pp. 49–67. JSTOR, www.jstor.org/stable/1127388.

17. https://www.parentingforbrain.com/authoritative-parenting/

18. https://www.healthline.com/health/parenting/authoritative-parenting#consequences

19. https://www.acpeds.org/parents/authoritative-parenting

20. https://www.verywellmind.com/what-is-authoritarian-parenting-2794955

Psychology and Division of Mental Health and Wellbeing, University of Warwick, Coventry, UK:

Victims [of bullying] were at increased risk for displaying psychotic experiences at age 18 and having suicidal ideation, attempts and completed suicides. Victims were also reported to have poor general health, including more bodily pain, headaches and slower recovery from illnesses. Moreover, victimised children were found to have lower educational qualifications, be worse at financial management and to earn less than their peers even at age 50.[21]

Because long-term damage has been seen in adults who suffered from childhood bullying, my opinion is that there should be zero tolerance and even drastic measures taken to remove children from harm's way... including moving the child from the school to a safer one or even homeschooling for a while, if that's an option. Children are shown to recover more quickly if their safety is seen as a high priority by adults, and are taken seriously.[22] Imagine the impact it may have on you to be bullied now, even with all your adult coping mechanisms.

As we know from adult learning experiences, the major key to hyper-efficient learning is safety, passion and voluntary participation. In an ideal learning environment, the child should have the ability to feel totally safe while having the freedom to choose if they want to learn a particular subject out of genuine interest. This is one of the main tenets of Montessori education, which is *'designed to support the child's intellectual, physical, emotional and social development through active exploration, choice and independent learning.'*[23] If you cannot find a local Montessori or Steiner school, then it may be up to you to homeschool your child in the early years to give them the safest possible learning environment. Homeschooling is a huge commitment, to say the least. It may even involve moving to countries where homeschooling is legally permitted and financially feasible. This is one more reason to carefully consider the huge investment needed in having a child.

21. https://www.ncbi.nlm.nih.gov/pmc/articles/PMC4552909/
22. https://www.psychologytoday.com/us/blog/love-in-time-homeschooling/201003/bullying-reason-homeschool
23. https://www.nature.com/articles/s41539-017-0012-7

The Tribe Model

Another way to support and prepare for having children is to develop strong and deep connections with others in a geographically close community of like-minded people. Children seem to thrive in a supportive tribe-like living environment in which the parenting demand can be shared between many adults.[24] In my opinion, the nuclear family (two parents and kids under one roof) is not the ideal structure for raising children. Children seem to benefit from developing close relationships with a lot of different people, especially adults.[25] This requires the parents to maintain close relationships with other trusted adults.[26] This is a very rare setup in developed, first-world countries.

This concept of the tribe model in our modern society (also referred to as *tribal mapping*) is supported by the writings of tantric philosopher Alexander Bard:

People's individual differences [...] are connected to the fact that what survived (or not) in the Darwinian evolutionary process was not a few individual people but entire tribes – precisely in the capacity of entire tribes. Either they survived and procreated, or they perished. Thus it was the tribes with the most favorable collection and combination of properties at the time that survived, and the tribes that had the least suitable collective features that perished.

[...]

The tribe was every individual member's entire world, and also their life insurance policy – as long as one had both useful and practical skills to offer the collective that in return provided protection and fellowship.

[...]

The Swiss psychoanalyst Carl Gustav Jung calls these tribal roles archetypes. This means that all conceivable archetypes are present within the tribe's aggregate gene pool in order to optimize the tribe's chance of survival.

—Alexander Bard from his book *Digital Libido.*[27]

---

24. https://www.huffpost.com/entry/community-parenting-for-the-win_b_6918754

25. https://www.todaysparent.com/family/parenting/how-to-build-a-village/

26. https://pathwaysoffamilywellness.org/Parenting/why-children-need-community.html

27. Bard, A., Söderqvist, J. (2018) *Digital Libido—Sex, Power and Violence in the Network Society.* Futurica Media. ISBN 978-91-88659-96-5.

Another great point in this tribal mapping theory is that the distribution of majorities and minorities has remained constant throughout history and all the various forms of identities and sexual orientations play a beneficial role to the collective. The repartition is of the order of 92% heterosexual men and women, 4% androgynous types and 4% shamanic types. A good tribe needs all of these well-integrated and accepting of each other's roles. In the tribe, the androgynous types mediate between men (outer circle) and women (inner circle). The shamanic types mediate between tribes (they make rituals that bring tribes together). So these minorities have important roles, but while most people in the tribe will be fairly uncomplicated "men" and "women" who will have limited gender-fluidity. This set-up may provide an open-minded, inclusive and stable environment to bring up children in.

Motives

Even before conception, the first question you might want to ask yourselves is *'What are our motives for bringing another person into the world?'* Nobel laureates agree that overpopulation is one of the greatest threats to the Earth and animal species.[28] The earth doesn't seem to need more people on this planet. Decreasing population growth and higher infertility rates are seen as problems from a human economic perspective, but from the Earth's perspective, do we really need another few billion more people? Thus it might be worth carefully questioning our motives when the baby desire arises. In my perception, most people have children for unconscious reasons, or hidden motives. Here are some that really make me cringe:

- *'We're having a baby to try and keep our marriage together.'* (What a nice pressure to put on an incoming child!)
- *'It's just expected of me.'*
- *'It would make me feel complete!'*
- *'She really wants them, and I don't mind.'*
- *'Would be so nice to have someone to unconditionally need and love me.'*
- *'It sounds like fun. Why not?'*
- *'My parents want grandkids.'*

---

28. https://www.timeshighereducation.com/features/
do-great-minds-think-alike-the-the-lindau-nobel-laureates-survey#survey-answer

- *'I want to keep my genes going when I die.'*
- *'I'll get a government subsidy.'*
- *'Whoops!'*

My advice, if you ever hear yourself or your partner utter statements like that, then I would strongly suggest pulling your parenting buddies to one side and asking them what it's *really* like to be a parent. Ask for 100% honesty. They will almost certainly not want to be *too* honest, as it would make them sound like ungrateful parents, but do persist. Your ability to make an informed decision depends upon it. While having a highly conscious, undamaged child can be one of the most rewarding things in life, the opposite can be equally true and extremely stressful. The main factor in how damaged your child gets is of course you and your partner's self-development. Reality bites.

While there is the potential to raise very undamaged children (and potentially a whole new less-damaged society), I am not holding my breath that it will happen anytime soon (if ever). Maybe a crisis like the current COVID-19 outbreak may make people less judgmental and create a temporary hiatus on aggressive action against our neighbours, but humans do seem to have an incredible ability to become parochial and let subconscious envy take over even the most rational minds. It feels like loving thy neighbour when you see how badly people can behave is virtually impossible. It is certainly something I struggle with everyday. Baby steps.

Nevertheless, for my daughter's sake and the sake of future children, I pray this book may contribute in some small way to reduce the endless cycle of shame and misunderstanding we have around sex, and help with reducing the damage that it can make in society.

Full Circle

If you find yourself stuck at home and want to find a safe way to improve your life, there is plenty of homework in this book. Who knows, in a short time you might master these techniques and prove yourself a gifted sexual practitioner in ways that the world has rarely seen. I know the masculine loves a good competition and that is why I circle back to the tantric show-down. So guys, here's a little shopping list of boxes to tick if you really want to have a crack at the best tantric sex practitioner's crown:

- Master the techniques in opening a woman's body as covered in this book. De-armouring, g-spot squirting, cervix orgasm, womb orgasm and transcendent sexual states.
- Be able to reach the full tantric potential of the man's body, such as fully master the spasm reflex, only have a few mistakes per year and a fully de-armoured tantrically orgasmic ass (and be able to fully enjoy it as much as you naturally wish to).
- Regularly valley orgasm on the pudendal nerve. This is when you feel the intensity of the regular orgasm but without the spasm reflex. The prostate rhythmically slowly pumps, but not hard enough to forcefully ejaculate sperm, and thus allowing multiple double digit orgasms without the side-effects of the regular orgasm. It took me years to get to this, but you may be able to do that in a fraction of the time. But be patient, it's worth the work and incredibly pleasurable.
- Realise that physical sex is only a doorway into deeper transcendent states that are reflected in a deeper capacity to live functionally in daily life.

As I said at the start of this book, if you are willing and able to prove that you really are better at sex, I would love to hear and learn from you.

There are more levels of advanced sexual tantric practice but they are not for this book.

Onwards and upwards!

Photo credit: *Jill Wellington* (https://pixabay.com/users/jillwellington-334088/?tab=popular), https://pixabay.com/photos/youth-active-jump-happy-sunrise-570881/

POSTSCRIPT

Focus on the Teachings, Not the Teacher

Dear reader,

It means a lot to me that you made it all the way till the end of the 50 misconceptions. This book has been a labour of love, sweat and tears for the last 3 years. To have you read these words feels both intimate and vulnerable.

I've worked extensively with this unorthodox subject that is tantra since 2001. It's been a crazy, wild and enriching exploration with many ups and many downs. I never thought I would be able to put pen on paper and condense 2 decades of tantric sexual teachings into writing.

But here it is and I'm immensely grateful to you for reading my first book as an author. I also invite you to check out the Adult Bedtime Story in the next few pages as a last bonus.

After reading this book people may mistakenly think it would be cool to be me and maybe even emulate or copy me. Having been me much longer than anyone else, I can assure you that is not such a good idea. Sorting out your sex life is kind of like good dental hygiene. Brushing your teeth doesn't really make your life overflowing with pleasure and happiness, but *not* brushing your teeth will certainly make your life miserable in the not too distant future. Same with sex.

Who I envy is *you*, the *normal* person that can use these powerful skills and still fit into society. The tantrically skilled straight or hetero-flexible person that can wear gender appropriate clothing and be treated as someone that fits into the tribe. The person that can go home for Christmas to their family dressed the way they want to, or walk down the street without being pointed and laughed at, or in fear of being bashed. All the lucky, normal women that can find a nice successful boyfriend and not be treated like a sexual fetish and hidden behind closed doors in shame.

I'm not saying I'm a victim. Of course, every day I choose what I wear and how I live my life, but to me not being authentic is the slow, suffocating death of compromise.

POSTSCRIPT

So to you, my lucky reader, take these powerful and hard won teachings and enjoy applying them into your life, and watch yourself transform into the version that Nature intended you to be.

If you liked this book then please leave your review on Amazon or any other place you may have bought it. Share your review on social media and with your friends. By doing that you will be helping me spread the message of a more conscious tantric sexuality to new potential readers. I read every review the book gets and each of them means a lot to me.

So once again, thank you.

Alexa Vartman

APPENDIX
An Adult Bedtime Story

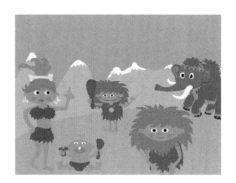

Once upon a time, in a land far, far away, there lived an unusually smart young woman called Yona. She, like many of the other animals, enjoyed sex as well as touching herself, especially in springtime when food was more abundant and life was less stressful.

The sex life of a caveman was very similar to that of the animals. Just like the other mammals, her brain was not developed enough to be able to masturbate to internal visual fantasies. The Homo Sapiens lived in harmony with the other species (unless they were eating them, of course), and enjoyed an innocent and simple life. Although they found their cousins, the Neanderthals, to be rather stupid (and they had such awful body-hair issues), they tolerated them... and even occasionally fornicated with them.

Then, one day, something unprecedented happened in Yona's brain. Unbeknownst to her, she was the first of her species to reach a tipping point in her neocortex evolutionary development, where she could create mental scenarios that had not yet happened. She could remember her little sexual escapade in the cave the night before, and also could project that image into an imagined future. Lo and behold, she found a new ability to make up all sort of arousing scenarios without any physical reality. She simultaneously discovered she could accentuate the fantasies by touching her clitoris at the same time.

After several months of nightly practice, she was surprised by an entirely new feeling. While rubbing her clitoris and fantasising, an intensely pleasurable spasm between her legs erupted, lasting for about 5 seconds. It felt like nothing she had ever felt before. Yona was unsure how to feel about this explosion that had occurred within her. Yes, it was pleasurable... but what was it? She had never heard anyone else describe this experience of fantasising and rubbing her clitoris to create that feeling. Was she the only one? Should she tell the others what she had discovered? Yona became fearful that this would make her different from the others, creating a separation between herself and her other cave homies. After all, considering the horrible words they used in reference to the hairy Neanderthals, she couldn't risk being too different. Yona decided it would be best to keep this new delight to herself, at least for now.

About the same time, she started to experience a new emotion that was not so pleasant. A strange little guilty feeling after each orgasm as if she was secretly doing something wrong. Thus, sexual shame was born in humans.

But the shame did not outweigh her enjoyment of cheap thrills... besides, she had already decided not to tell anyone about her little secret. Unknown to her, she had just invented a new skill which would prove invaluable... the ability to *deceive* others. She could enjoy her private sexual world in her head and still appear to be as innocent as the rest of the tribe, and therefore remain acceptable... her survival literally depended on it.

Unlike the other women in the tribe, Yona was now horny all the time and not just when the season dictated it. With much practice, she became accomplished at creating all sorts of wild fantasies. She could visualise 2 men, then 3, 4, 5... all fornicating with her at the same time! Before long, she was imaging the curvy cave girls joining in the party as well. Her cave mates had no idea what they were missing out on, but she certainly could not clue them in. Quite quickly, she became hopelessly addicted to rubbing her love button and simultaneously exercising and developing her visual and prefrontal cortex in the process.

Within a short period of time, her brain began to develop skills that none of the other Homo Sapiens could do. She developed the capacity to do very *good* things, like imagining scenarios in the future for planning... but she also *knew* how to do *bad* things, like tricking others. This gave her an extraordinary advantage over everybody else. For example, when a neighbouring tribe asked her, *'Hey, do you know where the buffalo are?'* Yona replied, cunningly, *'Take a right, then a left at the first tree past the termite mound, head straight into the desert and just keep going. Can't miss them. Big hairy things with horns.'* Thereby ensuring more meat for her own tribe.

Over time, she became more and more revered by the rest of the tribe due to her seemingly magical powers. She had the ability to plan for the future and also manipulate others to her will. Rather easily, she became the chief, enjoying a status of being seen as a magical goddess... but a goddess that knew both good and evil.

One day, she met her male counterpart. A chief from a neighbouring tribe called Ling. Her attraction not only revolved around his physical attractiveness but also his brain and intelligence matched her own closely. They became good friends, but he wanted to learn Yona's magic of being able to manipulate the future. Eventually, she decided to confide in him and share her little secret. She educated Ling on how to visualise past and future images for sexual pleasure enhancement.

After much practice, Ling grokked the technique and did something no other males of any species could do. He learned how to use his visual cortex to create a mentally-arousing fantasy while stroking his penis and learned to ejaculate outside of a vagina at will.[1] All of a sudden, he had acquired the ability to use his life-force creation energy purely for a short-term thrill.

Like Yona, Ling quickly became addicted to this new-found ability. Ling was also now fornicating with Yona more than ever, but sex and frequent masturbation was taking up a good portion of his time and consuming a lot of energy. In the beginning, Yona and Ling were having a lot of passionate sex. But after a few months, Ling's appetite for Yona began to diminish. Now, the other females in their newly-combined tribe started looking more attractive, and thus another new emotion was born... jealousy. Yona's response to this was to use her mental skills to control Ling to be in an exclusive sexual relationship with her, by means of creating endless emotional drama. The first pussy-whipping forced monogamy relationship of mankind was created. Now, there were frequent bouts of anger and greediness in Ling and Yona's cave. Oh, joy!

One of the most astounding effects of their new sexuality was that this couple could procreate all year round. Childbirth had been naturally restricted by nature by requiring that ovulation and the shorter breeding season coincide. But when Yona gave birth, there was a new problem that was rarely experienced in natural human birth. You see, up until that point,

---

1. Humans, like animals, have always been able to have the spasm orgasm, but apes don't seem to be able to fantasise, and rarely masturbate to orgasm. As we descend from apes, it seems only logical that there must have been an *'evolution'* and transition from apes to human masturbatory habits.

humans lived in an environment free from many of the mind-created problems and mental stress that Yona and Ling were now experiencing. The unnatural use of the prefrontal cortex for lying, jealousy, deceiving and drama was creating a kind of stress and hardness in her body. Combining this with frequently clenching the base of her body to create those pleasurable rhythmic contractions had caused her to harden the most vulnerable place in her body… her cervix. For the first time in human evolution, an artificially hardened cervix resulted in abnormal cervical pain during childbirth.

Ling was also experiencing his own problems. His excessive orgasming was creating an emotional rollercoaster. In the past, he had experienced only brief mood swings during the relatively short mating season, but now Ling was experiencing it daily. The hormone disruption after each ejaculation made him unusually grumpy, flat and ill-tempered, especially in relation to Yona. His flat mood made him crave the brief thrill of orgasm even more. Ling was quickly losing his child-like innocence, connection and ability to empathise with the others in his tribe. He tried to suppress his endless appetite for new women, but sexual thoughts occupied his mind for most of the time. Thus, the first eternally horny, hungry ghost-like man was born.

But the loss of innocence also had an upside. Yona and Ling became powerful leaders and rapidly expanded their tribe through their *'magical'* ability to create offspring at will. These traits were also being passed on to their children through their genes and upbringing. Their unusual brains had given them a competitive advantage, and more and more, they treated the rest of the tribe as ignorant slaves. The more they developed, the more they became isolated and could only relate to those able to think in the same way as they did. Within time, they would restrict their bloodline to those that could think in the same way as them, and thus the first royal family was born.[2]

Over time, they became more aggressive and hostile to those who were different. This was especially true with the vastly different Neanderthals. The Homo Sapiens ability to use their less intelligent tribe members as soldiers and plan attacks with strategic warfare allowed them to rapidly wipe

---

2. Perhaps there is some amusing parallel with the Bible as well and the scientific Mitochondrial Eve and Y-chromosomal Adam. In layman's terms, all people on earth seem to be related to one man and one woman that may have lived at roughly the same time when there were approximately 10,000 human inhabitants on the planet. https://en.wikipedia.org/wiki/Mitochondrial_Eve

out the physically stronger Neanderthal tribes within a few generations.

Eventually, they grew more disdainful of the simple ones. It was decided that anyone not related to them by blood would not be allowed to breed and would simply be worked to death. The master-race of nature-disconnected humans had begun.[3]

Photo credit: *Grafikacesky* (https://pixabay.com/users/grafikacesky-947552/), https://pixabay.com/vectors/prehistory-mammoth-family-1142403/

---

3. Humanity began when we evolved into efficient copying machines. This is how we can learn complex behaviour like speaking and so on. Unfortunately, this also led to mimetic desire: we want what others want. And that leads to conflict due to competition and ensuing envy end jealousy in the tribe. The way out of that conflict is to pick a (random) scapegoat and to release the tension in the tribe in an orgy of sexual violence. Then there's peace again until mimetic rivalry and tension rise again and another orgasmic, violent release is needed. This cycle of tension followed by violent, orgasmic release that goes on at the **level of the tribe** is reflected on the **individual level** in our human sexuality: tension followed by orgasmic release. Tantric practice aims at going beyond this tension and release cycle in an embodied way at the personal level. But in that way, it indirectly also strikes at the core of the global destructive tension and release cycle that plays at tribal level. (This footnote is thanks to a philosopher friend of mine who highly respects the work of René Girard and upon reading this bedtime story he sent me his philosophical analysis on it).

ABOUT THE AUTHOR

Alexa Vartman is the female version of Alex Vartman, born in Adelaide, Australia. She started meditating when she was 10 years old. Her deep intuition and constant inquiry on why humans are suffering, including herself, led her to a very introspective journey into tantra.

Since 2001 she has been traveling all around the world, studying and exploring tantra extensively. She has researched different spiritual traditions and tantric lineages (such as Buddhism, Hinduism, Christianity, Taoism etc...), fully immersing herself in these practices to live and integrate them on physical, emotional, mental and spiritual levels.

In 2010 Alexa founded the school The New Tantra. She has conducted hundreds of speeches and workshops in over 15 countries. She has a knack for developing tools to make modern tantric practices accessible for Western minds of the 21st century. Her work has helped thousands of people improve their sex lives and lead happier and better functioning lives.

Alexa has bridged tantra with other fields such as psychology, philosophy and science, making the insights that are depicted in this book highly effective, accessible and powerful. Her ideas are easy to understand and can be practised by anyone who desires to change their current patterns and ideas.

This book is a result of her research and deep insights over the last decades. It invites us to look at sexuality and experience it in a totally different way. It offers a gateway into a new sexuality for humanity. By dealing with our sexual conditioning, we can live more playful, innocent and happier lives for ourselves and for the future generations to come.

For speaking engagements (and potential boyfriends/hot versatile transexual lovers :-)), please send me a message through the contact form on www.50misconceptionsofsex.com.

Photo credit: *Jan Dahlqvist, Asfalt Communication AB*

Because future editions of this book are constantly updated for optimality and relevance, we are able to correct, update references and add useful quotes and new scientific insights. Please send them through the contact form on www.50misconceptionsofsex.com.